7 Steps to a Healthy Brain

Think Younger, Look Younger, Feel Younger

Paul Winner, D.O., FAAN

Clinical Professor of Neurology

Nova Southeastern University

Fort Lauderdale, Florida

Director, Premiere Research Institute

Director, Palm Beach Headache Center

at Palm Beach Neurology

www.DrWinner.org

7 Steps to a Healthy Brain

Copyright © 2008 by Dr. Paul Winner

Visit us on the Web at: www.DrWinner.org

Apex Solutions, LLC

Lulu Publishing

This book is available at special discounts for bulk purchases for sales promotions or premiums. Special editions, including personalized covers, excerpts of existing books, and corporate imprints, can be created in large quantities for special needs. For more information, write us at Contact@DrWinner.org

Book Images done by Clayton Bowen, Eagle Lake, Texas.

ISBN – 13: 978-1-4357-1068-9

Additional Books authored by Dr. Paul Winner

Headache in Children and Adolescents.

Headache in Children and Adolescents. 2nd ed. 2008.

Headache and Migraine in Childhood and Adolescence.

Young Adult and Pediatric Headache.

A Note to the Reader

Preface

You can do this!

The sole purpose of this book is to help you live longer and live better. As a neurologist, I have developed a program to achieve better Brain Health, by revealing the secrets to optimum brain function and by utilizing straight-forward solutions on how to keep you and your brain young. The goal of this book is to assist the reader to both capitalize on an opportunity to maintain a healthy brain; as well as, to help prevent many of the neurological disorders that affect us as we get older. This book will guide you in a straight-forward, direct and practical manner to help maintain your brain at full function for as long as possible.

It has become clear that there is not going to be a single pill that will ultimately achieve this goal and by taking that into consideration I found it is necessary to develop a comprehensive seven step approach. This book is also designed to help those who are already afflicted with neurological disorders. Hopefully, we can help them to help themselves in relieving migraine and back pain, giving some concepts to address issues of memory loss, Alzheimer's, degenerative diseases of the brain, problems with sleep disorders, neurovascular issues such as stroke and other neurovascular concerns.

I would like to take this opportunity to thank my friends and colleagues who have been so encouraging with regard to the development of this text. Specifically I would like to thank Tracy J. Simkowitz, Scott Turner, and Clayton Bowen for their help in getting this book to print. I would also note that this work could not be possible without the instruction and guidance of my former professors and my many colleagues in research and education, locally and nationally.

In addition, I am indebted to the team of assistants who helped in the preparation of this material. Finally, I would like to thank my family: my parents for always being so encouraging, my wife for always being so patient and supportive, and my children and the patients who provide inspiration.

Dr. Paul Winner

Introduction

The deterioration of brain function is noticeable in some individuals as young as thirty. It has been said that this is just normal, inevitable aging of the brain. If this is true, how do we explain patients in their 70's and 80's who have the brain function of individuals in their late 20s? Therein lies the key issue.

The good news is that the majority of us do not have to experience progressive brain degeneration. There are steps that we can take against this brain degeneration.

We have yet to discover a single magic pill that will reverse the aging process. Certainly, our environment and our genetics play a key role in how we age. However, there are certain factors that we can control that will give us the best chances of aging well. There are seven steps that we can implement immediately to maintain a healthy brain and body in order to live a longer and better life.

These seven imperative steps outline how you can maintain a healthy brain throughout your lifetime in a practical, clear and concise manner. If we utilize these steps properly, we may overcome some of the obstacles presented by genetics and environment. It is imperative to understand that these seven steps will not only help you maintain a healthy brain, but these steps may also help you live a better life.

This book will take you through the key concepts to implement in your life so that you can maintain a healthy brain and stay young. Your time to start is now.

Think Younger,
Look Younger,
Feel Younger.

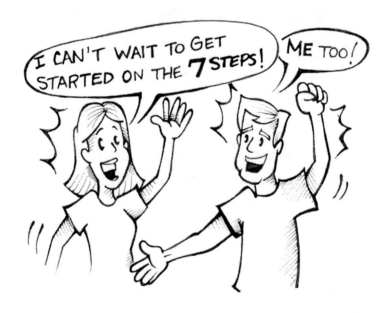

Table of Contents

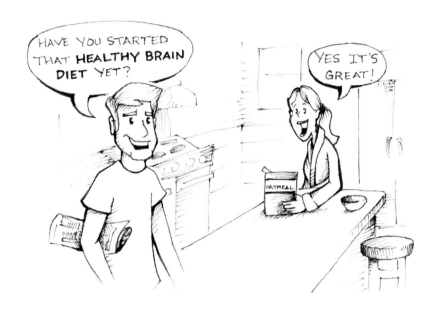

Step 1: Healthy Brain Nutrition

Nutrition and the Brain

The brain is the most complex organ in our body. It utilizes the most energy of any organ in the human body, requiring roughly 20% of the entire body's energy supply to function normally. The brain consists of more than one hundred billion nerve cells. Medical research clearly shows the important role of nutrition in maintaining a properly functioning neurovascular and cardiovascular system. Which nutrients are the most important for maintaining a healthy brain? We will discuss this issue and give you some practical examples of good choices to help maximize lifelong brain vitality.

The four basic nutrients your body needs are fats, carbohydrates, proteins, and water. A proper diet requires a balance of foods that contain essential fatty acids. These include Omega-3 fatty acids which primarily come from fish, seafood, and a variety of dark green and other colored vegetables. Complex carbohydrates are found in whole grains and nuts. Proteins can be obtained from lean meats, poultry, fish and vegetables. Additionally, remember to add appropriate supplementation with a focus on antioxidants. These are all vital and necessary to maintain a healthy brain and to prevent premature aging of nerve cells. Let us take a look at these nutrients in detail. (Balch, 2006)

Fats

> **The Doctor Says...**
> Your brain is roughly 60% fat.

Your brain is roughly 60% fat. It is imperative for optimal brain health to supply the body with appropriate nutrients, including certain fats on a daily basis. Fats come in more than one form. The saturated and trans fats (these are fats that are solid at room temperature), over time, can result in significant damage to the brain, cardiovascular and neurovascular systems. You want to limit your intake of saturated and trans fats. Some examples of foods containing these fats are cheeses, margarines, butter, and many baked goods. Fortunately, today it is easier to avoid trans fats due to proper labeling. Trans fats should be avoided at all cost. They clearly have a negative impact on a healthy brain. Trans fats elevate the risk for stroke and heart attack mostly by blocking blood flow and promoting inflammation, both of which can be deleterious to the brain and lead to premature aging. (Balch, 2006)

Good fats like Omega-3 and Omega-6 fatty acids are essential for proper brain and nerve cell function. However, the ratio of these fats is also important. Omega-3 fatty acid is primarily found in fish and seafood, but can also be found in certain vegetables and in items such as flaxseed, walnuts, and soy bean oils. Eggs fortified with Omega-3 fatty acids are widely available, and are a good source of this important nutrient.

> **The Doctor Says...**
>
> Good fats like Omega-3 and Omega-6 fatty acids are essential for proper brain and nerve cell function.

Omega-3 is an anti inflammatory and is actually composed of two key elements, DHA (Docosahexaenoic acid) and EPA (Eicosapentaenoic acid). These fatty acids are important in maintaining proper brain function. DHA is important for brain development, learning, and prevention of cognitive decline. Additionally, DHA is important for structural framework of the nervous system, specifically the nerve cells. It is also notable that the DHA anti-inflammatory component inhibits the cytokines, particularly interleukin-1, beta and TNF Alpha, which appear to impair cognitive function and can potentially lead to significant damage to the neurovascular and cardiovascular systems. EPA is critical as an anti-inflammatory and is vital for communication between nerve cells.

Omega-3 fatty acids are vital for optimum brain function, structure, development, and signaling of nerve cells. Omega-6 is also important for proper function, but if taken in too high a quantity, it can actually promote inflammation and oxidative stress free radical formation, exactly what we are trying to avoid. It is a fact that the brain is not fully developed until roughly age 25, and continues to require maintenance throughout adult life. Thus, Omega-3 fatty acids and Omega-6 fatty acids are vitally important to maintaining a healthy brain.

Omega-6 fatty acid is found in sunflower, corn oil, sesame seed, peanut butter and to a lesser extent soybeans, walnuts, and flaxseed. Too much Omega 6 can actually be potentially detrimental: if consumption of Omega 6 is 10 to 20 times greater than Omega 3, it can lead to inappropriate levels of inflammation. The ideal ratio is 1:1 Omega-3 to Omega-6 fatty acid consumption.

Most individuals can obtain Omega-3 fatty acid through supplementation of fish oils, a relatively inexpensive way of obtaining this vital nutrient. It is important to obtain supplements from a high quality manufacturer who has appropriate filtration systems and takes precautions to avoid exposure to mercury and other

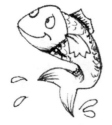

toxins that can be present in the fish and seafood from which the oil is obtained. Some of the newer formulations are also better tolerated by patients, making it easier to continue the utilization of this product. These Omega-3 fatty acids can also be consumed in their natural state by eating fish and seafood. Some good choices are Spanish mackerel, wild salmon, sardines, anchovies and herring. These fish are some of the highest quality sources for EPA and DHA. Spiny lobster, halibut, shrimp, catfish, sole and cod do contain some EPA and DHA as well. Thus, it is important to vary your diet and consume fish of different types about twice a week. (Logan, 2006)

A cautionary note: there are concerns about the mercury content in larger fish such as tuna and swordfish. Mercury, heavy metal, PCB and other toxins found in large fish can possibly result in detrimental effects to a developing fetus or even to the developed brain of an adult. It is best to limit consumption of these fish to about once every two weeks, and for pregnant women to avoid them entirely. Thus, for these individuals, it is suggested that they consider supplementing their diet with the Omega-3 supplements that are available. I urge you to obtain them from a quality company that has addressed these concerns in their manufacturing process.

It has been stated that DHA can help maintain significant cognitive function and memory, even in the face of potential onslaught, as in early Alzheimer's and early dementia complex. Clearly, further studies in this area will help to address this issue in greater detail. Can Omega-3 fish oils be important in childhood learning, in helping to control attention deficit disorder, or even Alzheimer's? Again, research needs to address these issues.

Omega-3 can also be found in buffalo meat at high levels, in the compound form called alpha-linolenic acid. Foods such as mayonnaise are being made with canola oil bases to increase levels of "good fats" in everyday items. Eggs enriched with Omega 3, as I mentioned earlier, are a good source of an anti inflammatory food. Thus, the proper eggs can be very beneficial in your diet. Eggs also supply other nutrients including choline, which is important in the structural components of brain cells, specifically phospholipids. (Logan, 2006)

Truly, Omega-3 fatty acids are super nutrients for a healthy brain. High levels of Omega-3 are associated with improved cognitive function and improved longevity. Our goal is to slow the aging process down; Omega-3 is a key component in our "fountain of youth."

Complex Carbohydrates

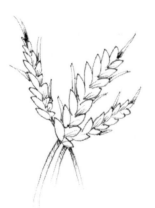

Complex carbohydrates provide a consistent source of energy for the brain and the body. They consist primarily of whole grains. Some examples are oat bran, whole wheat and brown rice. Cereal grains are often a very simple and easy way to obtain complex carbohydrates.

However, not all cereals are created equal. It is important to read the labels and make sure that the cereal grains you are consuming do not have inappropriate amounts of sugar or high fructose corn syrup. These are the carbohydrates you neither want to consume, nor intermix with your complex carbohydrates. Carbohydrates that come from processed sugars such as candy bars and soft drinks do not provide the highest quality energy source; they actually have the potential to increase the risk of diabetes, cardiovascular disease, and neurovascular disease. In fact, long-term excessive use can result in increased insulin secretion, and elevated insulin, or hyperinsulinemia. Many doctors feel that this is a risk factor for the development of neurodegenerative diseases such as Alzheimer's Disease. (Balch, 2006)

Proteins

Protein is essential for the proper development and maintenance of the human brain and the human body. It provides energy and is essential in the manufacturing of enzymes, antibodies, hormones, and in tissue maintenance. Amino acids are the building blocks for all proteins. There are essential and non-essential amino acids. Essential amino acids need to be consumed; non-essential amino acids can be produced throughout the body from the essential amino acids. It is relatively easy to obtain dietary amino acids from food sources such as meats, poultry, fish, dairy products, eggs, and milk.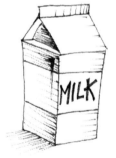

A Note for Vegetarians and Vegans

It is difficult to obtain all of the complete proteins necessary in a diet primarily from vegetables. If you choose to obtain your proteins from vegetables, it is important to use combinations of certain vegetables in an effort to obtain all of the essential amino acids necessary for proper maintenance of muscle tissue and the building blocks for hormones, antibodies, and enzymes as needed. If proteins are consumed through grains, legumes, and leafy green vegetables, it is important to consume a variety of these. For example, if a person is to consume beans, it is important to add nuts, corn, or wheat to that meal. If a person consumes primarily a substance such as wheat, it is also important to add other components such as rice, nuts, or seeds in an effort to obtain all of the essential amino acids.

Thus, it is important to have a varied diet with the proper amounts of the various food groups so that one can obtain all of the essential amino acids on a daily basis. For most individuals in the United States, this is not a concern. The issue actually is the consumption of too much protein. Thus, it is important to have appropriate portion size and to utilize an appropriate dietary menu to obtain what is necessary without over consumption (Balch, 2006)

A good source of protein often overlooked in the U.S. is that from soy bean products, such as tofu and soy milk. They contain the complete essential amino acids necessary, as well as other vital nutrients like vitamin-B6.

Finally, yogurt is also a very good source of complete protein necessary in our diets. As an added benefit, yogurt contains vitamins A and B-complex. It is advisable to utilize protein that does not have added sugars and flavors, so buy unsweetened organic yogurts and add your own fruits or flavors as you desire. (Bowden, 2007)

Water

Water is essential in every bodily function as we are primarily made up of water. It is important to drink an adequate amount of safe drinking water daily. Try to consume water that is properly filtered to remove potential toxins. Water is vital in the proper transport of nutrients and waste products in the body. How much water should you drink daily? You should drink about six, 12 ounce glasses per day. This could vary according to your activity level and the time of year.

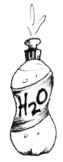

Free Radicals vs. Antioxidants

Let us focus a moment on the importance of addressing free radicals. Free radicals are substances that are released in your body by the breakdown of certain substances like polyunsaturates. Free radical production can lead to damage of delicate nerve cells. Free radicals damage fat and protein substances in the brain. Most concerning is the potential damage to DNA, the basic building blocks of all human beings.

The good news is that when our bodies are given the proper nutrients, we develop an excellent defense against the creation of free radicals. There is not one single compound or food source that can build and maintain a healthy defense system on its own. A balanced intake of nutrients and supplements that we will discuss can result in the optimum control of free radicals and increase longevity and healthy brain function. Also, simply limiting our intake of items that contain sugar and high fructose corn syrup can go a long way. Low levels of chronic inflammation are also a significant enemy to healthy brain function. Therefore, it is important that we consume natural anti-inflammatory compounds. ***A good example of an anti-inflammatory compound is the wild blueberry.*** This fruit is an excellent source of a dietary antioxidant that helps preserve cognitive function due to its high quantity of phytochemicals. Although blueberries are not powerful enough to prevent dementia, they clearly seem to assist in preserving memory. Natural sources of antioxidants are found all over the world. In the United States, it is relatively easy to obtain wild blueberries or farmed blueberries.

Many fruits, vegetables, and herbs, other than blueberries, are good sources of antioxidants. Many contain phytochemicals, important compounds that act as powerful antioxidants; for example, anthocyanins are found in high quantities in blueberries and cherries, isoflavonies are found in soy, flavonols in apples, and catechins in teas such as green tea. Other key antioxidants are beta-carotene, lutein, lycopene, and zeaxanthine. Sources of beta-carotene include carrots and other orange vegetables. Lutein is often found in green vegetables such as broccoli. Red vegetables like tomatoes and red peppers contain lycopene. Finally, zeaxanthine is found in vegetables such as corn and spinach, the yellow/green 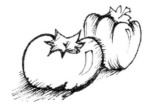 vegetables. It is important to eat a variety of these vegetables and fruits in your diet; be sure to obtain the freshest vegetables possible. If at all possible, avoid canned vegetables; use fresh or frozen organic vegetables. Always try to obtain the original fruit, if at all possible, or organic fruit juice that does not have added sugars or high fructose corn syrup. Certainly, it is best to avoid soft drinks, which are excessively high in sugars and artificial coloring. (Pizzorno, 2006)

Added supplements containing B complex vitamins are also exceedingly important; in particular, riboflavin is felt to have beneficial effects in the prevention of migraine. (Winner, 2008) Riboflavin can be obtained naturally in fortified cereals, nuts, wild salmon, halibut, and certain leafy vegetables such as broccoli, spinach, and asparagus. The B-vitamin complex is also vitally important to help cognition, memory enhancement, brain function, longevity and alertness. (Bowden, 2007)

A four to six ounce glass of wine is equivalent to one serving. Men will benefit from consuming one to two servings per day. Women should consume only one serving per day to reap the maximum benefits. The researchers at the University of California, at

Davis tested a variety of wines to determine which types had the highest concentrations of flavonoids. They determined that the wines with the highest flavonoid content were: Cabernet Sauvignon, followed closely by Petit Syrah and Pinot Noir. Both the Merlots and the Red   Zinfandels were found to have less flavonoids. White wines had an overall smaller amount of flavonoids than the red wines. It would seem that the sweeter the wine, the lower the amount of flavonoids. So, stick to the dryer red wines, they are your best bet for a flavonoid boost. Obviously, wine needs to be consumed in moderation. It is the red grape that has the antioxidant component, and thus purple or red grape juices are probably just as good a choice. (Cooper, 2004; Pizzorno, 2006; ynhh.org)

The theme is clear: there is a need to have a balanced, varied diet and to make intelligent choices. For example, given the option of choosing steamed broccoli or French fries, it is clear that the steamed broccoli is the proper choice to maintain a healthy brain. In all fairness, occasionally having French fries over the course of someone's life will probably have no real significant detrimental concerns, but to have it in abundance is not the best choice. You may find the book: "The 150 Healthiest foods on Earth", by Dr. Jonny Bowden, a helpful guide in giving you more ideas for healthy choices.

Micronutrients: Vitamins and Minerals

There are many other nutrients that are vital to proper brain function. The brain requires proper amounts of magnesium, which is vital for communication between nerve cells. Magnesium can be found in oat bran, wheat, brown rice, nuts, and leafy green vegetables.

Selenium is also important for brain health, and is vital to other organs. Selenium is a potential brain antioxidant that can be found in nuts, seafood such as wild salmon and Halibut, and whole grains.

Zinc helps metabolize Omega-3 fatty acids. It seems to help with attention and focus, and can be found in grains such as oatmeal, beans, nuts, and some lean meats.

Folic acid and vitamin-B12 are essential. Deficiencies of vitamin-B12 can cause serious neurologic disorders, which can be confused with dementia complexes, peripheral neuropathy, and depression. Good sources of vitamin-B12 include lean meats, eggs, dairy products such as milk, wild salmon and some other seafood. Folic acid is also important for proper brain and cardiac function. It can be obtained primarily in fortified cereals, but it is also in green vegetables, beans, and wild rice.

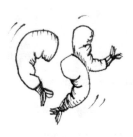

Vitamin-D is important for attention and alertness, and is felt to influence motivation and enthusiasm. It is vitally important for proper metabolism. Vitamin-D can be obtained through seafood such as wild salmon, sardines, and shrimp. It can also be obtained in bee pollen, cheese, spinach and fortified milk.

Vitamins C and E, especially when combined with beta-carotene, form very powerful dietary antioxidants that help optimize brain function. Vitamin C can be found in citrus fruits, bee pollen, carrots, cabbage, Goji berries, Acai, Noni, grapefruits, grapes, guava, lemons, oranges, raspberries, green peppers, tomatoes, potatoes, cauliflower, beets, broccoli and asparagus. Good sources of Vitamin E are seafood, spirulina, almonds, almond oil, walnuts, sunflower seeds, peanuts, pecans, sesame seeds, avocados, leafy vegetables, soy, wheat germ, whole grains, palm oils and beef.

Anti-Inflammatory Compounds

Anti-inflammatory compounds are very important in maintaining a healthy brain. Inflammatory conditions seem to not only be involved in arthritis, but also seem to be involved in cardiovascular disease, diabetes, obesity, and possibly even neurovascular disease. As such, it is important to consume compounds that have anti-inflammatory effects for proper brain function.

Anti-inflammatory components can be found in naturally occurring compounds such as ginger, green tea, and turmeric (curcuma longa) that is found in curry. It would seem that they protect the mitochondria (the ingredient in your cells that produce energy) from damage and may actually have protective powers for prevention of dementia.

Ginger has been used for countless centuries in an effort to control GI (gastrointestinal infection) and headache symptoms. Ginger is very flavorful and has a clear anti inflammatory and antioxidant component.

Green tea, which has become very popular in the United States, contains several antioxidants and significant anti-inflammatory properties, while also being a very pleasant drink. It is also found to inhibit bacteria. More research is clearly needed to explore the benefits of this wonderful drink. Clearly, it can be used as a substitute for sugary soft drinks. It may also have some benefit for controlling cognition and prevention of various chronic neurological disorders such as Alzheimer's. Green tea may turn out to be a very friendly brain drink!

> **The Doctor Says...**
> Green tea, which has become very popular in the United States, contains several antioxidants and significant anti-inflammatory properties, while also being a very pleasant drink.

Coffee has a significant potential as a source of antioxidants. One or two cups a day helps with focus and may 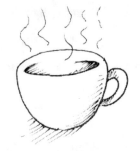 prevent degenerative changes of the brain. Moderation is the key and it is important not to exceed more than 16 ounces per day, otherwise dependency issues and potential detrimental side effects may become apparent. As with anything, too much of a good thing can turn out to be a problem! (Logan, 2006)

As we address issues of proper food intake, it is also important to address the quality of our food. We need to spend time learning to look for the best source of our food products, usually organic or frozen foods are preferable. (Figure 1) When you can, try to avoid canned foods and foods with added salt, which are often unnecessary as part of our general diet.

Figure 1

<u>Natural Foods</u>- these foods are minimally processed and contain no artificial colors, flavorings, or preservatives.

<u>Organic Foods</u>- the U.S. Department of Agriculture (USDA) strictly enforced proper production of these foods by using the following categories:

- "100 Percent organic"- products included all organically produced (raw and processed) ingredients (excluding water and salt).

- "USDA Certified Organics"- made with 95 percent or more organic ingredients.

-"Made with Organic Ingredients"- foods may include 70 to 95 percent organic ingredients.

- Foods made with less than 70 percent organic content can include the organic ingredients on the ingredient label.

Body Mass Index (BMI)/ Waist Management

It is important that we try to maintain our body mass index (BMI) between 18 and 24.9. BMI 25 to 29.9 is considered overweight and BMI 30 and greater is considered obese. For how to calculate your BMI, go to Figure 2.

Figure 2

Body Mass Index (BMI)

Standard (Pounds)

$$BMI = \frac{\text{Weight in Pounds}}{(\text{Height in inches})^2} \times 703$$

Standard (Kilograms)

$$BMI = \frac{\text{Weight in Kilograms}}{(\text{Height in meters})^2}$$

Go to www.7StepstoaHealthyBrain.com to have your BMI calculated for you in the "Reader Resources" section. BMI tables are also available on this website.

If you are overweight or obese, you should strongly consider going on a diet today. Which is the best diet? The best diet for you is the one that you will keep. There are a myriad of diet plans available to choose from. Please review the reference section of this chapter for some suggested diet texts that you may find helpful. It is best to review this with your physician or allied healthcare professional.

The management of our waist is important because it is an indicator of how much omentum fat we have. The omentum in someone with a normal BMI tends to have a fine mesh of small fat molecules internally overlying the abdomen. As our BMI increases, this mesh becomes a carpet and eventually takes on a mass that is typical of what we see with an extended abdomen. We know that stress contributes significantly to the development of omentum fat and thus an increased waistline and increased BMI. I refer you to the chapter on stress management for some suggestions on how we can control our stress in a positive manner and ultimately help to control our food intake.

I wish I could say that the problem we have with obesity is only in adults in the United States, but it is unfortunately now involving our children, adolescents, young adults, and older adults. It has essentially become an epidemic that is spreading even beyond the United States. It is imperative that we get a handle on appropriate food intake.

The impact of pediatric obesity and headache is presently being evaluated. Adult studies have shown a correlation between obesity and headache. The Pediatric-Adolescent Section of the American Headache Society demonstrated a trend of obesity with increased headache frequency and disability. Recently, 913 consecutive patients at 7 centers were evaluated and 19.6% were found to be obese and 36.5% at risk or obese. During the routine headache management, nutritional impact on headaches including weight control was discussed with all patients. Subsequent follow-up information was obtained from 213 patients at ~3 months and 174 patients at ~6 months from 4 centers. In the total population, the mean age was 12 years, mean weight - 50 kg, mean height – 150 cm, and mean BMI - 21.5. The mean headache frequency per month was reported to be 12.

At 3 months, 14.6% were obese and at 6 months 15.6% were obese. At 3 months, those obese or at risk patients that reduced their BMI had a significantly greater reduction in their headache frequency and disability compared to those with weight gain. These reported differences continued to increase at 6 months for those that reduced their BMI. Thus an elevated BMI is significantly correlated with disability, suggesting a combined contribution to disability. The impact of obesity and headache in the pediatric population needs further study; clearly, in those at risk or obese that were able to reduce their BMI, there was a greater degree of improvement in headache frequency and disability. (Hershey, 2007)

There is an increasing amount of data showing that there is risk to the brain due to obesity. This omentum fat results in increased inflammation, free radical formation, hypertension, symptoms of stroke, depression, cognitive interference, dementia, diabetes and Alzheimer's disease.

Increased weight also leads to a lowering of self-esteem, a lower quality of life and shortens our life by years to decades. (Roizen, 2006)

Dr. Mehmet Oz, in his book "You On A Diet", very clearly addresses this issue. I highly recommend that you consider reading his book that focus on the issues of waist management. (Roizen, 2006)

It is noted that this increased abdominal girth due to omentum fat results in fat cells generating free radicals thus increasing oxidative stress. Also, the fat cells produce chemical messengers including Interleukin-6 (IL6) and TNF-Alpha which ultimately result in promoting inflammation and possibly contributing to altered mood, anxiety, and impaired cognitive function. Over a longer period of time, chronic elevations of these compounds may result in immune dysfunction.

It has been suggested that the use of antioxidants may help to reduce or counteract some of this negative effect. Most important is to lose the omentum fat.

Increased oxidative stress and inflammation have been observed in situations of increased BMI, consistent with obesity, morbid obesity, and the observations of anxiety, depression, and possibly even schizophrenia. Is it a direct cause and effect? That relationship still remains to be seen; research is necessary, but it is highly suggestive. Either way, there is enough data to reinforce the importance of obtaining a normal BMI in an effort to diminish cardiovascular and neurovascular disease. There have also been concerns of increased obesity resulting in increased risk of Parkinson's disease and dementia associated with Parkinson's.

Increased stress, resulting in increased cortisol levels and obesity, clearly seems to be detrimental to normal brain health. Chronic stress, contributing to an increased BMI, will ultimately lead to an increase in cardiovascular and neurovascular risk factors, diabetes, heart disease, stroke, dementia, and depression. Thus, it is imperative as part of good health strategies to address, control, and prevent chronic stress.

There are various ways to address this increased cortisol level. I refer you to the chapter on stress management in this book. Increasing the fiber in your diet, especially in the morning as part of your breakfast, may prove to be beneficial in lowering your stress and cortisol levels. Obviously, a comprehensive method of controlling your cortisol and maintaining an appropriate BMI of between 18 and 24.9 is necessary. More recent work has shown that higher fiber intake is associated with lower body weight and is important in maintaining a proper BMI. There is discussion as to what is the appropriate amount of fiber intake for men and women. It is suggested by Dr. Oz in his text, "You On A Diet", that the daily intake of roughly 25 grams of fiber per woman, and roughly similar amounts for men, is a good target zone. Other doctors have suggested even higher amounts of fiber approaching 35 grams a day for women. (Roizen, 2006)

The benefit of fiber is that it allows you to eat more and gives you a feeling of fullness. The importance is to choose the right fibers such as whole grains, fruits, and vegetables. Use those that have the most nutrition and the highest antioxidant

> **The Doctor Says...**
> The benefit of fiber is that it allows you to eat more and gives you a feeling of fullness.

properties. Suggested meal plans and recipes are listed at the end of this chapter to make it easier for you to enjoy a high fiber meal. (Tribole, 2007)

Choosing appropriate drinks such as green tea, water, and dilute organic fruit juices are far better choices than carbonated beverages containing high sugar or sweetened fruit juices. Also, avoid excessive amounts of caffeine, although small amounts may be beneficial.

Calcium is important as part of our proper diet, and interestingly enough, calcium intake late in the day may actually prove beneficial as part of your weight loss program. The average calcium intake varies anywhere from 500 mg to 1500 mg, depending on your diet and provided there are no significant deficiencies. Additionally, calcium taken in the evening may also help facilitate proper sleep. (Logan, 2006)

If you do have an elevated BMI, 25 or greater, it is important that you speak to your physician or allied healthcare professional and choose an appropriate weight loss program that fits your medical and your physiologic needs. Remember that fiber, calcium, and spices can be both enjoyable and helpful in assisting with weight loss. Do not forget to take the appropriate supplements and fortified antioxidants in an effort to help you control and prevent cardiovascular and neurovascular disease.

If you do have proper body weight, it is important that you eat the best food possible, get the best supplements possible, eat balanced meals, get appropriate exercise, and follow the seven steps to a healthy brain.

> **The Doctor Says...**
> It is important to remember the saying "seven foods for seven days".

It is important to remember the saying "seven foods for seven days". It is suggested that in your diet across the course of the week, or even during each day, to consume: blueberries, spinach, walnuts, tomatoes, oats, yogurt, and green tea. Just keep the saying in your mind every day for a proper diet. (Figure 3)

Figure 3

7 Foods for 7 Days
(Best to consume these foods everyday)

1. Blueberries or (Pomegranates, Acai berry [antioxidants])

2. Spinach or (Kale, carrots [beta-carotene])

3. Walnuts or (Salmon, sardines, olive oil [omega-3])

4. Tomatoes or (Watermelon [lycopene,Vit-C])

5. Oats or (Blackbeans)

6. Yogurt

7. Green Tea [Polyphenols, catechins]

The Healthy Brain Diet

The concept of the healthy brain diet can be used either to lose weight or to maintain your ideal body weight. It is important to maintain your BMI between 18 and 24.9.

If you have a body mass index that exceeds 24.9, it is important to address the issue of weight loss using either the concept we are about to review or any of the diet systems that your physician or allied healthcare professional feels is appropriate for you. The key is to adopt a way of eating and exercising that you can continue throughout your entire life, maintaining an ideal body weight. Do not get   discouraged if you fluctuate significantly, even if you have a hard time getting started or maintaining a dietary concept. You are not alone. The key is to never give up; continue even if you fail on a single meal or day. Forget about it, forgive yourself, and move on to the next meal. The next day, just try a tiny bit harder to achieve that goal.

The foundation of the healthy brain diet is based on a single meal concept. Each meal has to be thought through to be either protein based or carbohydrate based. When you plan each day's meals and snacks, it is important to understand a few basic concepts. If you choose a carbohydrate based meal, it will take roughly three hours to digest that food. If you choose a protein based meal, it will take about four hours to digest your food. If you were to significantly mix these foods, the digestion process takes much longer. An extreme example of mixing all different types of foods is Thanksgiving dinner. Everyone remembers after a very lovely Thanksgiving dinner feeling tired and listless, not only from the turkey, but from the combinations of different foods. It can take four to nine hours to totally digest the food eaten during such a significantly large meal. Thanksgiving is pretty much an exception, but you need to remember this concept. This concept also includes the importance of appropriate fat introduced into your diet, as this chapter has addressed earlier. How do we truly utilize this concept, how do you make these choices at home, in a restaurant, or with friends at a barbeque? Let us begin a more concrete discussion in this matter.

If you do have an elevated BMI and you are using this concept to actually lose weight, you also have to consider portion size. We are fortunate; we are born with a built in scale. Look at your hand, the width, the length and the depth of your palm: that is about the amount of protein that you should consume at any given meal; for the most part for the day. More than that is often unnecessary for the

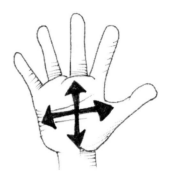

majority of average weight people. Look at the length, width, and depth of your fingers: that is about half the amount of vegetables to consume with that meal. This makes it relatively easy to figure out your portion size. We can be far more sophisticated in addressing this issue.

There are many diet companies and programs that have extremely sophisticated methods of determining portion size. If you feel more comfortable with such detailed methods, I encourage you to utilize that system. Many companies have addressed this and have done an excellent job. If you do not wish to address this portion size concept in such detail, this may be a simple way for you to make some decisions. Another way is that every time you have a choice between small, medium, and large, or between petite and regular in food choices; always choose the smallest size and the smallest possible portion. At some restaurants, this is not the best value for your money; however, it will be the best value for maintaining a healthy brain and a healthy body in the long run.

Breakfast

A simple breakfast is fruit. The right fruits deliver an immediate energy boost to your brain. It takes about 45 minutes to digest a banana or an apple; most other fruits take about 30 minutes.

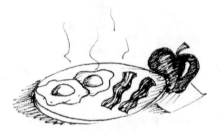

Some excellent choices for early morning brain energy include blueberries, raspberries, strawberries, peaches, plums, and pears. If you can, just get used to having fruit in the morning with a cup of coffee. Pick one of your favorite fruit juices, making sure that you are getting true 100% fruit juice without any added sugar or high fructose corn syrup. For example, 100% pure, organic cranberry juice is relatively low in sugar content naturally, containing only about 8 or 9 grams of sugar. In contrast, cranberry juice with a sugar content of 25 grams or greater contains added sweeteners, something you need to avoid.

It is important to educate yourself on the normal sugar contents of different juices; it is always best to buy organic whenever possible.

In general, the best fruits to consume in the morning are an apple or banana with a pear, peach, plum, apricot, melon or some berries. Every day, try to have a small cup of blueberries, blackberries, raspberries, strawberries or any type of berry that you enjoy. As with anything, use moderation with your intake of your fruit. Should you find that it is metabolized quickly, and within 1-2 hours you are really hungry, have a small (3-4 ounce) cup of blueberries, a peach, plum, pear, or apple. Try to avoid eating fruit about one hour before your scheduled lunch time: for most of us, this falls somewhere between 12:00 and 2:00 in the afternoon, so keep that in mind.

Oatmeal is another great choice for breakfast. There is a continuing discussion about the nutrient content of instant oatmeal. However, it still is a lot better than 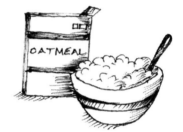 having two donuts or a buttered roll! Try to make your oatmeal with water, if you can, as opposed to added dairy products such as milk. If you are going to use milk, use fat-free milk (for an adult, there is no reason to consume fat in milk). To add flavor and help to decrease your appetite, add a little cinnamon to plain oatmeal. If you become extremely hungry a few hours after an oatmeal breakfast, a 4 - 6 ounce cup of a high quality, organic dry cereal makes an excellent mid-morning snack. Again, it takes roughly three hours to digest the carbohydrates, so it is important to time your snack so it does not influence your food choices at lunch.

Omega-3 fortified eggs are a good start to the day. Try to prepare your eggs without butter or margarine. A little olive or avocado oil can be used instead, and it is very flavorful. If you become extremely hungry a few hours later, I would suggest eating 3-4 ounces of walnuts or almonds at mid-morning.

Most people like to vary their choices, so have something different each day if you are one of these individuals.

Lunch and Dinner

Many cultures set aside enough time at lunch to have a relaxed, well prepared meal. Due to our busy schedules, many of us barely have 15-20 minutes to eat at noon. When possible, it is best for your health to try to focus solely on lunch. At lunch you have basically two main choices: a carbohydrate based lunch or a protein based lunch.

Protein Based Meal

If you choose the protein based lunch, your options include fish, poultry, or meat. Try to limit your intake of red meat, especially fatty red meats when at all possible. Again, look at your portion size. If you are at your ideal body weight, then you have already done this naturally or have figured this out over the years. If you are not, use the concept discussed earlier; eat portions the size of the palm of your hand for the proper intake of the protein.

With each lunch, I highly suggest you add a salad. Avoid adding ingredients that contain fat, including nuts, high fat dressing, and sugars (such as fruit). You can also mix all the different greens; dark greens are best, especially spinach.

If you choose to use a dressing try to pick one low in fat and calories. Here is a great trick: do not put dressing directly on the salad. Dip your fork in the dressing and then pick up your salad with the fork. You will use a lot less dressing this way! Another option is to use olive oil and vinegar. At all times you should be using Extra Virgin, First Cold Pressed Olive Oil. It is very important to do your best to get this type of an olive oil. Eat as much salad as you want, but limit the dress-

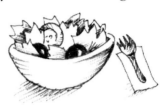

ing. Besides the salad, if you can, have a serving of steamed or raw vegetables. They can be seasoned, but avoid butter, margarine and excessive salt. It is best to choose vegetables that have a very low starch content when eating a protein based meal. These include green leafy produce such as spinach, broccoli, and string beans. If you are having steamed broccoli, you can eat as much as you want, which can help fill you up. Try not to eat to the point you are full; eat only until the feeling of hunger is gone. I know this seems ludicrous to most of us, but if possible, try to take 45 minutes to an hour to eat lunch.

Carbohydrate Based Meal

If you choose a carbohydrate-based lunch, you have a lot more options for your choice of vegetables. This is the time to have your potato, beans, and other starchy vegetables. You will find you really cannot eat that much of these vegetables because they are very filling. Again, use no butter or margarine, and very little salt. This is also when you can choose a pasta option, adding some bread if you see fit (preferable a multigrain). Add a salad, as discussed above.

It is now late in the afternoon. If you feel you want a snack (most people often do somewhere around 3:30 to 5:00), consider what you had for lunch and what you are planning for dinner. If you had a protein based lunch, have 3-4 ounces of walnuts, almonds or pecans. Make up your own mixture, but try to have raw nuts and avoid salt. This will lock you in to a protein-based dinner. If you had a carbohydrate based lunch and it is going to be 1-2 hours before you have dinner, you need to again have some dried cereal. This will prepare you for a carbohydrate based dinner. Sometimes I find that when I follow this regime it is easiest to plan my entire day's meals, choosing either a carbohydrate or protein based meal plan focus.

Carbohydrate Based Meal Day

For example, on a carbohydrate day, I may start the day with some oatmeal, have some vegetables and salad for lunch, and at dinner, some lentil soup and high quality bread. This is a good time to have a little spaghetti; the portion size of the spaghetti (pasta dish) is similar to that of the proteins, recall the idea of the palm of your hand.

Protein Based Meal Day

If I get up and decide that I am going to have a protein based meal day, then I would start the day with eggs. Lunch might be a small breast of chicken with some vegetables, and at dinner, I will often have fish and non-starchy vegetables with a very nice salad.

Fruit for breakfast is compatible with either a protein or carbohydrate day. I happen to be a fruit lover, so I pretty much have fruit every morning, but occasionally, when traveling or visiting, my options are limited.

Dessert is always a temptation. There are some basic dessert rules. Most importantly, avoid butter and margarine at all costs. This is a challenging situation. If you are trying to lose weight, desserts should be avoided until you obtain a BMI between 18 and 24.9.

Fruit at the end of a meal is metabolized differently; therefore, we do not receive the full benefit from these nutrients. Fruit is much, much better taken in the early part of a meal, preferably 30-45 minutes prior to the meal. Many European meals start with a little fruit (often melon) about 30 minutes prior to the first course. Night time snacks should be based on dinner: dry cereals for a carbohydrate based dinner and nuts for a protein based dinner. Avoid the cakes, cookies and ice creams that are so prevalent in today's society.

Once you have reached your ideal body weight and have learned how to regulate portions, a small portion of a rich dessert is certainly something you can enjoy!

The issue of dairy is a bit complicated. Cheeses, for instance, contain significant amounts of fat, yet they can be a good source of protein. It is important, especially when you are trying to lose weight, not to completely remove cheeses in your diet, but to limit them somewhat; make them more of an "accent" than a central part of a meal. Also, avoid cream sauces when at all possible; they have a very high fat and calorie content. That said, it is quite reasonable to use fat-free milk as a protein choice. Also, yogurts are excellent and a good part of a protein meal. This will be a little easier to understand when you review the Healthy Brain Diet – Sample Meal Plans, that actually have some more detailed concrete examples of how to set up meal plans over the course of several days.

Restaurants and Eating Out

The Doctor Says...
Become proactive and request the steak NOT be cooked in butter or margarine products, nor have any salt added.

These same options can be exercised when in a restaurant. This requires a little bit of creativity and discussion with restaurant staff. For example, a steak is often served with French fries or baked potatoes, and vegetables with butter or cheese sauces. It is here where you have to become proactive and request the steak NOT be cooked in butter or margarine products, nor have any salt added. You may also request that vegetables (spinach, broccoli, or string beans) be steamed or prepared with olive oil. Also, ask that you receive a double portion of vegetables (spinach, broccoli, or string beans) instead of a potato. Most restaurants are happy to comply with these requests.

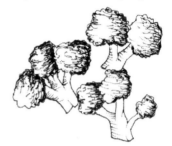

The healthy brain diet cannot be accomplished by dealing with food issues only. In order for this diet to be successful, whether in dietary mode or maintenance mode, it is imperative to exercise. There will be more about exercise in a later chapter, but know that you must exercise, preferably at least five to six days a week, for 30 minutes to one hour each day. If you cannot do this, at least go for a walk for at least 20-30 minutes every day. Some experts recommend taking at least one day off, a quite reasonable request, but at least six days out of the week, one should go for a nice long, brisk walk. If you have not exercised in a long time and if you are significantly overweight, I highly recommend that you review this with your physician or an allied healthcare professional. They can be immensely helpful and guide you to the diet and exercise plans that are most appropriate for you. Remember, the key is to do something to get your BMI between 18 and 24.9. Then do the other steps in conjunction with nutrition in order to maintain a healthy brain.

7 Day Healthy Brain Meal Plan

A 7 day sample Healthy Brain Diet is listed so that you can actually begin today. Future correspondence will give you additional information and insights into this concept of a Healthy Brain Diet.

Day 1
A Protein Based Meal Day

Breakfast
- Organic 100% cranberry juice.........................6 to 8 oz
- Egg omelet (Omega-3 or organic eggs) with   vegetables (tomato, mushrooms, spinach, broccoli)
- Coffee or herbal tea.

Morning snack (if needed)
- Shelled walnuts... 3 to 4 oz

Lunch
- Mixed salad topped with cooked turkey, grape tomatoes, and cucumbers, with Italian vinaigrette (on the side).
- Herbal tea or water

Afternoon Snack (if needed)
- Celery stalks filled with peanut butter or 3 to 4 oz shelled walnuts.

Dinner
- Spinach salad with toasted sliced almonds and tarragon vinaigrette (on the side).
- Shrimp in a garlic marinara sauce with cooked mushrooms and served with chopped flat leaf parsley.
- Herbal tea or water

Evening Snack (if needed):
- Shelled walnuts...3 to 4 oz

Day 2
A Carbohydrate Based Meal Day

Breakfast
- Organic 100% blackberry juice.........................6 to 8 oz
- One minute cooked oatmeal and powdered cinnamon. If preferred, add skim milk, almond milk or soy milk.
- Coffee or herbal tea.

Morning Snack (if needed)
- Dry cereal...6 to 8 oz

Lunch
- Broiled veggie burger topped with low fat cheese, lettuce and tomato.
- Roasted red bell peppers with extra virgin olive oil and vinegar.
- Salad and/or any vegetable of your choice
- Herbal tea or water

Afternoon Snack (if needed)
- Baked tortilla chips...4 oz

Dinner
- Salad with boiled green beans, boiled red potatoes and boiled sweet onions with extra virgin olive oil and fresh lemon juice or vinegar.
- Manicotti filled with spinach and ricotta cheese topped with a light marinara sauce.
- Fresh early green peas sautéed in extra virgin olive oil
- Chopped onion with chopped basil.
- Herbal tea or water.

Evening Snack (if needed)
- Dry cereal...6 to 8 oz

Day 3
A Mixed Meal Day

Breakfast
- Organic 100% apple juice................................6 to 8 oz
- Toasted 7 grain or whole wheat bread with organic preserves and/or cereal with skim milk.
- Coffee or herbal tea.

Morning Snack (if needed)
- Dry cereal...6 to 8 oz

Lunch
- Chef salad with red leaf lettuce and low fat blue cheese dressing (on the side).
- Herbal tea or water

Afternoon Snack (if needed)
- Shelled Walnuts..3 to 4 oz

Dinner
- Chicken piccata with white wine, capers, fresh squeezed lemon juice and garnished with lemon slices.
- Boston lettuce leaves and raspberry dressing (on the side).
- Steamed broccoli
- Herbal tea or water.

Evening Snack (if needed)
- Shelled walnuts..3 to 4 oz

Day 4
A Mixed Meal Day

Breakfast
- Organic 100% pomegranate juice....................6 to 8 oz
- An apple or banana served with fresh blueberries, straw-
berries or raspberries.
- Coffee or herbal tea.

Morning Snack (if needed)
- Fresh blueberries, strawberries or raspberries (eat at least
30 minutes before lunch).......................................1 cup

Lunch
- Light tuna salad with chopped celery, onions and relish
topped with fresh lemon juice and flat leaf parsley.
- Romaine hearts of lettuce and sliced tomatoes.
- Herbal tea or water.

Afternoon Snack (if needed)
- Mixed nuts (eat at least 4 hours before dinner)....3 to 4 oz

Dinner
- Mixed green salad.
- Baked ziti with eggplant, mushrooms and tomato sauce.
- Green beans cooked in chopped garlic and served with
extra virgin olive oil.
- Herbal tea or water.

Evening Snack (if needed)
- Dry cereal..6 to 8 oz

Day 5
A Mixed Meal Day

Breakfast
-   Organic 100% orange pineapple juice..............6 to 8 oz
-   Waffle with cinnamon and preserves, if desired.
-   Coffee or herbal tea.

Morning Snack (if needed)
-   Dry cereal..6 to 8 oz

Lunch
-   Garden vegetable soup...1 cup
-   Salad greens and vegetables (tomato, mushrooms, spinach, broccoli, or string beans), topped with chicken breast and raspberry vinaigrette (on the side).
-   Herbal tea or water.

Afternoon Snack (if needed)
-   Mixed nuts (eat at least 4 hours before dinner)....3 to 4 oz

Dinner
-   Salad with red leaf lettuce topped with asparagus spears, and French dressing (on the side).
-   Meatless chili with vegetables, chopped veggie burger, and kidney beans.
-   Spinach cooked in chopped garlic and extra virgin olive oil.
-   Herbal tea or water.

Evening Snack (if needed)
-   Dry cereal..6 to 8 oz

Day 6
A Protein Based Meal Day

Breakfast

- Organic 100% cranberry juice.........................6 to 8 oz
- Poached eggs with or without vegetables (tomato, mushrooms, spinach, or broccoli).....................2 to 3 eggs
- Coffee or herbal tea.

Lunch

- Mixed salad greens with vegetables (tomato, mushrooms, spinach, broccoli, or string beans) and topped with broiled shrimp and raspberry vinaigrette (on the side).
- Roasted red bell peppers with extra virgin olive oil and vinegar.
- Herbal tea or water.

Afternoon Snack (if needed)

- Mixed nuts..3 to 4 oz

Dinner

- Beets and sweet sliced onions with Italian vinaigrette.
- Broiled or poached wild salmon with olive oil based dill sauce.
- Spinach cooked in chopped garlic and extra virgin oil and topped with toasted pine nuts.
- Mixed salad with dressing of your choice (on the side)
- Herbal tea or water.

Evening Snack (if needed)

- Mixed nuts..3 to 4 oz

Day 7
A Carbohydrate Based Meal Day

Breakfast
- Fresh squeezed orange juice..............................6 to 8 oz
- An apple or banana served with fresh blueberries, straw-berries or raspberries.
- Coffee or herbal tea.

Morning Snack (if needed)
- Fresh blueberries, strawberries or raspberries (eat at least 30 minutes before lunch).......................................1 cup

Lunch
- One minute cooked oatmeal and powdered cinnamon. If preferred, add skim milk, almond milk or soymilk.

OR
- Broiled veggie burger topped with low fat cheese, lettuce and tomato.
- Roasted red bell peppers with extra virgin olive oil and vinegar.
- Salad and/or any vegetable of your choice.
- Herbal tea or water.

Afternoon Snack
- Baked tortilla chips..4 oz

Dinner
- Pasta with a tomato sauce.
- Mixed salad with dressing of your choice (on the side).
- Any vegetable of your choice along with boiled green beans, boiled red potatoes and boiled sweet onions served with extra virgin olive oil and fresh lemon juice or vinegar.
- Herbal tea or water.

Evening Snack (if needed)
- Dry cereal...6 to 8 oz

SUMMARY

It is important to have a properly balanced diet. Pick a variety of richly colored fruits and vegetables. Buy organic whole grains. Get organic foods. Try to eat fish at least twice a week (be careful of the larger species such as tuna and swordfish, which should be consumed much less frequently). Herbs such as

The Doctor Says...

Pick a variety of richly colored fruits and vegetables. Buy organic whole grains. Get organic foods. Try to eat fish at least twice a week

garlic, parsley, basil, and oregano are useful both as antioxidants and to give flavor to food.

United States Food Pyramid

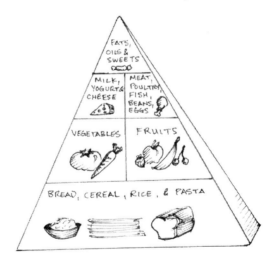

Recently, the United States has adopted a new food pyramid and clearly it is an improvement, but I suggest that you look into the food pyramids of other countries, specifically the Asian food pyramid. It seems to be closer to where we want to be to have a healthy brain.

For example, one meat dish is only consumed monthly; one poultry dish and an egg dish may be eaten weekly. And you may indulge in sweets only occasionally.

Asian Food Pyramid

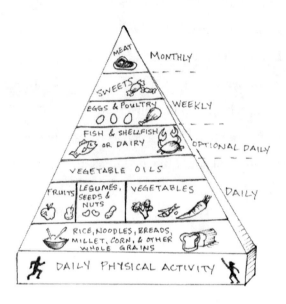

References and Recommended Reading

Balch PA. Prescription for Nutritional Healing. 4th ed. New York, NY: Avery Penguin Group; 2006. pp3 - 807.

Bowden J. The 150 Healthiest Foods on Earth. Gloucester, Mass: Fair Winds Press; 2007. pp8 - 324.

Chopra D. Alternative Medicine. 2nd ed. Berkeley, CA: Celestial Arts; 2002. pp557 – 938.

Cooper KA, Chogram, Thurnham D. Nutrition Research Reviews. June 2004. 17(1):111-129.

Greene B. The Best Life Diet. New York, NY: Simon & Schuster; 2006. pp2-267.

Hershey Ad, Kabbouche MA, Winner P, et. Al. Obesity in Pediatric Headache Population: A Multi-center Study. Oral Presentation at the 49th Annual Scientific Meeting of the American Headache Society, June 7-11, 2007. Chicago, IL.

Hobbs C, Haas E. Vitamins for Dummies. Hoboken, NJ: Wiley Publishing, Inc.; 1999.pp1-318.

Logan AC. The Brain Diet. Nashville, Tennessee: Cumberland House; 2006, 2007. pp1-277.

Null G. The Complete Encyclopedia of Natural Healing. New
    York, NY: Kensington Books; 1998.pp3-712.

Page L. Healthy Healing 12th ed. Healthy Healing, Inc.; 2004. pp289-
    623.

Pizzorno JE, Murray M. Textbook of Natural Medicine. 3rd
    ed. St. Louis, Missouri: Churchill Livingstone
    Elsevier; 2006. pp709-2201.

Roizen MF, Oz MC. You on a Diet. New York, NY: Free
    Press; 2006 pp3-354.

Schnur S. The Reality Diet. New York, NY: Avery, The Penguin
    Group; 2006, 2007. pp1-397.

Skidmore-Roth L. Mosby's Handbook of Herbs & Natural
    Supplements 3rd ed. St. Louis, Missouri: Elsevier Mosby;
    2006.pp1-923.

Tribole E. The Ultimate Omega-3 Diet. New York, NY: McGraw
    Hill: 2007. pp1 -324.

Ulbricht CE, Basch EM. Natural Standard Herb & Supplement

Reference. St.Louis, Missouri: Elsevier Mosby; 2005. pp22-789.

Winner P, Lewis DW, Rothner AD. Headache in Children and Adolescents 2nd ed. Hamilton,Ontario:BC Decker, Inc.; 2008 pp1-314.

YNHH.org/online/nutrition/advisor/red_wine.html

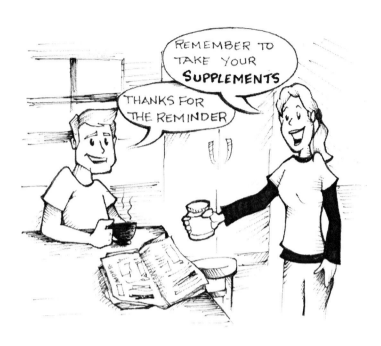

Step 2: Healthy Brain Supplements

It is a fact that many of the foods we consume today do not contain the nutrients they once did, even in the best organic form we can obtain. This leaves our body void of many of the essential building blocks that it needs to continually function on a high level. There is only one way to give our body the full complement of nutrients and vitamins that it needs, through supplementing. It is imperative to include the highest quality supplements as part of your daily routine.

> **The Doctor Says...**
>
> ...many of the foods we consume today do not contain the nutrients they once did...

> **The Doctor Says...**
> As with food products, not all supplements are created equal.

As with food products, not all supplements are created equal. Most are not independently tested and may have high quantities of unnecessary and /or potentially dangerous ingredients. You want a supplement that used the highest quality ingredients and does not contain sugar, artificial sweeteners, flavors, coloring or preservatives. Ideally, a high quality supplement should not contain milk, eggs, peanuts, crustacean shellfish, soybeans, tree nuts, wheat, yeast, or gluten. It is important that you study the labels and research your supplements in order to obtain the highest quality supplements.

This chapter is broken into two parts. The first part discusses an overview of the supplements that you should be taking as they may

> **The Doctor Says...**
> The first part discusses an overview of the supplements that you should be taking...

be considered in the management of General Brain Wellness, Migraine and Headache, Memory Loss, Pain, Stroke, and Sleep. Everyone should read the General Brain Wellness section of Part 1. These are supplements that everyone should be taking on a daily basis to keep their brain functioning at full capacity. If you suffer from Migraine/Headache, Memory Loss, Pain, Stroke, or Sleep, please refer to the section that you are most affected by. Your respective section will help to give you specific directions on how to most effectively supplement and best improve your daily life.

As we discussed before, it is difficult to find supplements of the highest quality. I am currently working with other physicians to help fulfill this need. Please visit www.DrWinner.org for updates on these highest quality supplements.

Part 2 is a comprehensive review of the effects that each individual supplement has on your body. This is for more advanced users and should be used as a reference. If you would like to understand the specific influences of one specific vitamin or supplement use Part 2 as your reference.

Note: As always, please consult with your doctor and/or allied healthcare professional before beginning any supplements.

Part I: Your Supplement Guide

A) Healthy Brain Wellness / Longevity and Vitality

Everyone should start their day with a high quality multivitamin and a dose of Omega-3 purified fish oil. High concentrations of Omega-3 essential fatty acids are found in our brain and are important in the transmission of nerve impulses, brain development and normal brain function. (Balch, 2006)

It is important that the Omega-3

> **The Doctor Says...**
>
> High concentrations of Omega-3 essential fatty acids are found in our brain and are important in the transmission of nerve impulses, brain development and normal brain function.

fish oil contains the proper relationship of EPA (eicosapentaenoic acid) and DHA (docosahexanoic acid). Omega-3 essential fatty acids in fish oil inhibit the development of atherosclerosis; thus decreasing the risk of ischemic heart disease, reducing the risk of coronary heart disease (CHD) and neurovascular disorders. On February 8, 2002, the US Food and Drug Administration (FDA) announced it would permit the appearance of "consumption of omega – 3 fatty acid may reduce the risk of coronary heart disease (CHD)" on the labels of omega - 3 fatty acid supplements containing a dosage of EPA and DHA of up to 2000mg per day. It is important to consume adequate amounts of the highest quality Omega-3 essential fatty acids on a daily basis in an effort to prevent both neurovascular and cardiovascular disease. (Pizzorno, 2006)

The proper testing and processing of Omega-3 purified fish oil is necessary to remove detectable levels of heavy metal, dioxins and PCBs.

In order to assist in retarding the aging process Coenzyme Q 10 (CoQ10) and high quality B complex vitamins are important additions to maintaining a healthy brain.

Caution Diabetics:

Persons with diabetes should not take fish oil supplements before consulting with their physician or allied healthcare professional, because of their high fat content. They should discuss with their physician or allied healthcare professional how to obtain the proper amount of essential fatty acids from their diet and/or with the use of supplements.

B) Migraine / Headache

Migraine is a genetically inherited disease (non-contagious) with variable expressions of disability throughout the individuals lifetime. There are many pharmacologic and non-pharmacologic management options. An effective integrated approach for the treatment of a migraine/headache individual will combine traditional pharmacology with supplements and, when needed, physical therapy and/or behavioral therapy. One of the easiest parts of the integrated approach to initiate is appropriate supplements targeted for the migraine/headache sufferer. The rationale for the use of supplements is rooted in the present understanding of the mechanism for migraine, the hyper excitability of the migraine brain. Triggers such as low ionized magnesium levels, abnormal neuronal membrane ion channels, and abnormal energy metabolism can be targeted by supplements such as magnesium, riboflavin, vitamin C and coenzyme Q10 to help reduce migraines. Butterbur is an herb that may function as an anti-inflammatory agent to potentially prevent migraine headaches. (Winner, 2008)

> **The Doctor Says...**
>
> An effective and integrated approach for the treatment of a migraine/headache individual will combine traditional pharma-cology with supplements and, when needed, physical therapy and/or behavioral therapy.

Consider utilizing a high quality supplement with chelated Magnesium, Riboflavin (B-2), Vitamin C, and Coenzyme Q10 to address the increased disability associated with migraine headaches.

C) Memory Loss

The prevention of memory loss: as well as, addressing Minimal Cognitive Impairment (MCI), should include high quality supplements. Supplements to be considered include: Vitamin C, Vitamin E, Omega-3 purified fish oil (DHA), Vitamin D, Ginkgo biloba, Huperzine, Vinpocetine, Bacopa, Acetyl-L-Carnitine, Phosphatidylserine,and CoQ 10.

> **The Doctor Says...**
>
> The prevention of memory loss: as well as, addressing Minimal Cognitive Impairment (MCI), should include high quality supplements.

DHEA is also mentioned as a supplement to help retard memory loss. It is a hormone that needs to be monitored very specifically. You need to address how it is formulated. Let your doctor know you have added this supplement since this is a hormone.

Caution: DHEA should be avoided in males with prostatic hypertrophy as well as a history of prostate cancer and avoided by women with a history of breast cancer. Additionally for women, concerns of estrogen alteration need to be reviewed with their physician or healthcare professional should this be added in a supplement form.

When DHEA is utilized, it is important to consider the addition of other antioxidants such as Vitamin C and E. Also, Selenium can be used in an effort to prevent some of the potential toxic effects on the liver. One of the ways to limit some of the potential side effects is to utilize the formulation of 7 Keto DHEA, which is not converted into estrogen or testosterone, and thus would have less of an adverse event profile.

Should a patient already have early to moderate Alzheimer's dementia, additional adjustments of their dosing may be considered.

D) Pain

Over 75 percent of adults will be affected by back pain during their life, most often involving the lower back. It can be either acute or chronic and for some, both. Supplements can play an important part of both an acute and chronic management plan. (Balch, 2006)

Utilize a high quality targeted supplement with adjustments of chelated magnesium, adjustments of vitamin C, and the addition of glucosamine sulfate/Methylsulfonylmethane (MSM).

Considerations for calcium supplementation may also be necessary depending on the person's medical history and status as it pertains to their condition.

Should there be an acute exacerbation of back pain, the supplement DL-Phenylalanine may be considered as well. This is a supplement that is recommended for short-term use during acute pain exacerbations.

Caution: DL-Phenylalanine should not be taken by pregnant women or patients who are suffering from diabetes, hypertension, who have a history of melanoma (skin cancer), concerns with regard to anxiety, panic attack or generalized anxiety disorder or social anxiety disorder. Additionally not for patients who have difficulty with the metabolism of phenylalanine (PKU –phenylketonuria). Should there be any concern about whether this supplement should be taken, review this with your physician or allied healthcare professional before beginning supplementation.

IMPORTANT INFORMATION:

For persons who are taking Headache/ Migraine or Back Pain supplements, once symptoms are under control, revert back or begin the use of a Healthy Brain Wellness approach for primary supplementation. This is because one may no longer need the extra supplementation. Should symptoms of Headache/Migraine or Back Pain return, you should return to your specially focused supplements again.

E) **Stroke (Cerebral Infarction) / TIA (Transient Ischemic Attack)**

Stroke ranks first among all neurological disorders in frequency and importance in adults since it results in acute disability. It accounts for 50% of neurological disorders in a general medical center. (Victor, 2001) The key is to prevent this devastating disorder. Targeted supplements can play a pivotal role in prevention.

> **The Doctor Says...**
> Stroke ranks first among all neurological disorders in frequency and importance in adults since it results in acute disability.

Consider utilizing a high quality targeted supplement with chelated magnesium, CoQ10, adjustments of Vitamins C, E, B-6, B-Complex, and Omega 3 purified fish oil.

Caution for persons on anti-platelet or anticoagulation therapy:

Vitamin C, when taken with anti-platelet or anticoagulant therapies, can result in adverse events including GI or intestinal ulcers and can interfere with the desired therapeutic function of the anti-platelet agents Aspirin, Clopidogrel or [aspirin/dipyridamole], and blood thinner agents, like Warfarin. It is important that you review this issue with your physician or allied healthcare professional. Should you be taking any medications to help prevent the neurovascular and/or cardiovascular diseases of stroke or heart attack, you should restrict yourself to a minimal amount of this vitamin supplement, since large amounts can result in adverse events or possible injury.

Vitamin E when taken in conjunction with anticoagulants (Warfarin-blood thinner) or anti-platelet agents (Aspirin, Clopidogrel, [aspirin/dipyridamole]), consider using a lower dose range of 200 IU per day. Before starting Vitamin E added supplementation, I recommend that you review this with your physician or allied healthcare professional, and that they monitor this issue as needed. Persons who are taking medications in the prevention of stroke or heart attack (or both) will need to address this key issue with regard to their supplement usage and their overall health program.

General Cautions:

Supplements may be taken as part of a comprehensive and enlightened health program to help maintain a healthy brain, as well as to support healthy bodily functions. Supplements added to any medical regime should be reviewed with your physician or allied healthcare professional, especially for patients who are taking anti-stroke medications. Should you be taking aspirin, Clopidogrel or [aspirin/dipyridamole] or anticoagulation protocols, such as Warfarin, you may need to have the supplements and the medicines you are taking monitored for potential interactions (adverse events that could occur). Remember that supplements, although not normally given as prescription medications, are indeed beneficial, but can cause side effects and potential interactions.

F) Sleep

There are many items that contribute to poor and inadequate sleep. Though, one of them should not be the improper supply of vitamins and minerals. B-vitamins are vital to the body control of tryptophan and other amino acids that are a necessity for proper sleep. Oftentimes, our behavior such as increased alcohol intake, smoking or other environmental factors, can reduce our intake of the B-vitamins. Thus, it is important to consume adequate quantities of vitamin-B3 niacin which is important in the regulation and the effectiveness of tryptophan. *There is some suggestion that adequate amounts of vitamin-B3 will limit and reduce insomnia for those who suffer from this disorder.* Vitamin-B3 is also important to avoid depression. It may also be important for blood sugar control and for just general proper sleep. Remember, when we are sleeping, we do not eat and thus we are able to affect proper weight management. Vitamin-B6 is important in the production of serotonin which has far reaching importance as a vital neurotransmitter. Vitamin-B12 is necessary for normal sleep patterns and may also help to avoid or limit insomnia. (Breus, 2006)

> **The Doctor Says...**
> Vitamin-B12 is necessary for normal sleep patterns...

The B-vitamins can be obtained in your diet in whole grains, broccoli, nuts, cereals and various vegetables such as potatoes. (Bowden, 2007)

A deficiency of Folic acid can cause insomnia, thus it is vital that adequate amounts of folic acid are consumed daily. There is also a notation that folic acid, depending on the form, may not be as absorbable in about two-thirds of the population, thus it is important for you to understand whether you absorb the standard folic acid products or not. (Breus, 2006)

Calcium is, as we previously discussed, important; it can be very helpful if taken late at night to aid in sleep and for its calming effect on the nervous system. As we have discussed, doses of 500 mg to 1500 mg are optimum and can be given across the day. Often,

> **The Doctor Says...**
>
> Calcium can be very helpful if taken late at night to aid in sleep.

magnesium is given in conjunction to calcium. ***Magnesium also has been shown to be important to assist in the prevention of poor sleep patterns***, and possibly to assist in the control of insomnia. Zinc deficiency has been linked to insomnia, so it also needs to be regulated. The issue of copper and iron may have some validity in regard to concerns of restless leg syndrome (RLS). If you do suffer from RLS, it is important that you review this with a physician or allied healthcare professional, since there are medical treatments that can be used in conjunction with supplements to control these symptoms. (Breus, 2006) It is important to address the presence of a sleep disorder and construct a comprehensive management plan.

Consider utilizing a high quality targeted supplement with appropriate B-vitamins, Folic acid, Calcium, Magnesium, and Zinc.

Part II: Supplement Review

Individual descriptions for each of the supplements

Multivitamin

A good multivitamin is the essential foundation for your daily supplements. Today, specific vitamins have been designed for men and women, addressing the special needs of each. It is imperative to take a high-quality multivitamin daily. Many of the foods we consume today do not contain the nutrients they once did, even in the best organic form we can obtain. It is imperative to include the highest quality supplements as part of your daily routine; I cannot stress this enough.

> **The Doctor Says...**
> A good multivitamin is the essential foundation for your daily supplements

Omega-3 Fish Oil

Fish oil is a superb source of Omega-3 essential fatty acids abundant in eicosapentaenoic acid (EPA) and docosahexaenoic acid (DHA). Sardines, salmon, herring, and mackerel have a higher content of Omega-3 factors than we traditionally know of with regard to fish such as cod. It is important to consume adequate amounts of the highest quality Omega-3 essential fatty acids on a daily basis in an effort to prevent both neurovascular and cardiovascular disease. (Pizzorno, 2006)

Every single living cell in our bodies contains essential fatty acids and they cannot be made by our bodies. ***Essential fatty acids reduce the risk of blood clots, reduce blood pressure, lower triglyceride and cholesterol levels, and improve our skin and hair.*** High concentrations are found in our brain and are important in the transmission of nerve impulses, brain development, and normal brain function. Essential fatty acid deficiency can result in memory loss and impair learning. Omega - 3 essential fatty acids are known to have cardioprotective effects, and prevent brain cell damage. (Balch, 2006)

> **The Doctor Says...**
> Essential fatty acid deficiency can result in memory loss and impair learning.

The EPA and DHA in fish oil inhibit the development of atherosclerosis, thus decreasing the risk of ischemic heart disease and reducing the risk of coronary heart disease (CHD). Fish oil can help reduce the risk of sudden death from a cardiac arrest. On February 8, 2002, the US Food and Drug Administration (FDA) announced it would permit the appearance of "consumption of omega – 3 fatty acid may reduce the risk of coronary heart disease (CHD)" on the labels of omega –3 fatty acid supplements containing a dosage of EPA and DHA of up to 2000mg per day. This has been done in an effort to help reduce the incidence of sudden death from a heart attack. Fish oils containing EPA and DHA have been found to suppress inflammatory mediators found in individuals with psoriasis and rheumatoid arthritis. (Pizzorno, 2006)

It is important that you obtain Omega-3 Fish oil that has been properly tested and fractionally distilled to remove detectable levels of the dangerous toxins: mercury, arsenic, lead, cadmium, PCBs, dioxins and other heavy metals.

Caution Diabetics:

Patients with diabetes should not take fish oil supplements before discussing this with their physician or allied healthcare professional, because of their high fat content. Patients should review the issue of how to obtain the proper amount of essential fatty acids from their diet, and integrate the use of supplements.

Vitamin B Complex

Vitamin B complex is vital in maintaining a healthy nervous system and a properly functioning brain. It also has importance in the maintenance of our skin, hair, liver, and eyes and is also important in proper muscle tone of the gastrointestinal tract (GI tract). ***Vitamin B complex is essential in energy production.*** The B vitamins are vital to proper brain function; a deficiency of Vitamin B12 plus B complex can present signs consistent with Alzheimer's dementia and thus without proper evaluations, could be misdiagnosed. It is more important to prevent such an event from taking place by having proper supplementation of B complex vitamins on a daily basis

> **The Doctor Says...**
> Vitamin B complex is vital in maintaining a healthy nervous system and a properly functioning brain.

as part of your diet. It is felt that the sublingual form, as well as the spray forms, are more easily absorbed and therefore a better choice, especially for older adults. B complex vitamins are generally felt to be nontoxic. The only exception is vitamin B3 niacin, depending on dosage. If not properly titrated, higher dosages can cause symptoms of nausea, vomiting, abdominal cramps, diarrhea, flushing and sometimes more severe interactions. If you are taking niacin, please review this with your physician or allied healthcare professional as part of your general health maintenance. (Pizzorno, 2006)

Thiamin (Vitamin B-1)

Thiamin (Vitamin B-1) is important for nervous system and appropriate cognitive function. This compound is also important with regard to our immune response, and aids in carbohydrate utilization for energy production. Thiamin can be depleted in the body from smoking, heavy metal pollutants, excessive sugar intake, stress, alcohol overuse and use of foods that are lacking in thiamin supplementation. Deficiencies of this compound can result in fatigue, confusion, memory loss, and insomnia. In rather severe cases, deficiency can result in beri-beri which is induced by chronic alcoholism and the lack of proper dietary intake of thiamin. Thiamin deficiencies have also been felt to be associated with various forms of Alzheimer's like dementias.

> **The Doctor Says...**
> Thiamin deficiencies can result in fatigue, confusion, memory loss, and insomnia.

When thiamin is taken in extremely high doses, it may potentially cause a harmful effect such as an upset stomach. Although, most would conclude that it is a relatively harmless compound even at higher doses.

Age itself may actually be a risk for thiamin deficiency and thus it is important to address appropriate supplementation of thiamin in our diet. Clearly, the concern is that of having difficulties with regard to cognitive function or issues as it relates to mental attitude and mood disorders. These disorders are adversely affected by lack of an appropriate amount of thiamin in our diet. Physical activity also places an added burden in increasing our thiamin intake, as does any added stress. (Pizzorno, 2006)

Riboflavin (Vitamin B-2)

Riboflavin, vitamin B-2, is part of the B complex vitamins. In some individuals when given higher doses, it has been found that they can control or at least decrease the number of headaches, specifically migraine. (Silberstein, 2008)

> **The Doctor Says...**
> Riboflavin B-2 can decrease frequency of headaches, specifically migraine.

This was first shown by Dr. Schoenen in 1988 where he had done a comparison of riboflavin versus placebo and was able to show a significant superiority of the riboflavin. In this case, 400 milligrams was used against placebo. (Winner, 2008) Riboflavin is also important in other aspects. It has been shown to be beneficial in some individuals for carpal tunnel as part of their treatment algorithm when it was combined with vitamin B6, which is Pyridoxine. When extra supplementation of these vitamins (B2 and B6) is used, once the person has controlled their symptoms, they should be discontinued because large doses for large periods of time could have adverse side effects such as interfering with antibiotic function. Also note that the B vitamins, specifically riboflavin, are easily destroyed by light, alcohol and some antibiotics. (Logan, 2006)

This vitamin can be found in fish, grains and cereals, broccoli, asparagus, spinach, yogurt, dairy products, milk and cheese. (Bowden, 2007)

Riboflavin is recommended to begin at 200 milligrams daily and then increased as tolerated by 200 milligrams in 7 days to a target dose of 400 milligrams daily, or less as tolerated.

Vitamin B-3 (Niacin or Nicotinic Acid, Niacinamide or Nicotinamide)

Vitamin B-3 is important for proper neurovascular and cardiovascular function. This compound is important to the nervous system, skin, and in the metabolism of carbohydrates, fats, and proteins. Thus, Vitamin B-3 is involved in many biochemical processes as they relate to energy and lipid metabolism.

Niacin is felt to lower serum levels of low-density lipoprotein (LDL) and triglycerides, while increasing the levels of high-density lipoprotein (HDL) cholesterol, thus potentially improving circulation. It has also been considered for use to help in the treatment of schizophrenia, other mental illnesses, rheumatoid arthritis, and as a memory enhancer. (Balch, 2006) (Pizzorno, 2006)

> **The Doctor Says...**
> Vitamin B-3 is important to the nervous system, skin, and in the metabolism of carbohydrates, fats, and proteins.

Symptoms of niacin deficiency may include: dementia, depression, dizziness, fatigue, headaches/migraines, insomnia, muscle weakness, skin eruptions/sores, diarrhea and loss of appetite.

Vitamin B-3 can be found in beef livers, brewer's yeast, eggs, fish, milk, nuts, pork, broccoli, cheese, tomatoes, wheat germ, whole wheat produces and some herbs (alfalfa, cayenne, chamomile, hops, and peppermint).

Some individuals experience a harmless flushing (vasodilatory) effect after taking the Niacin form of vitamin B-3. This effect does not occur when the Niacinamide (amide) form is used. But, the Niacinamide form is felt not to have all the properties of niacin. It is not felt to be effective in lowering LDL cholesterol. (Balch, 2006)

Caution:

Large doses of niacin (>1000 mg) have been associated with symptoms of diarrhea, nausea, stomach pain, itching, and cardiac arrhythmias.

Niacin is contraindicated in individuals with diabetes, since it can raise blood glucose levels. Individuals with gout, liver disease, peptic ulcers, or glaucoma should use caution when using niacin supplements. Women who are pregnant should also discuss this with their physician or allied healthcare professional, if they want to take niacin supplements. (Balch, 2006)

Vitamin B-6 (pyridoxine)

Vitamin B-6 pyridoxine is important in both the maintenance of brain and general physical health. Vitamin B-6 is vital for the nervous system to function normally. It also has properties to assist with the immune system, and it is important in the prevention of atherosclerosis, thus preventing stroke and heart attack. Its role with regard to the regulation of homocysteine (amino acid in the blood) as part of a combination of medicines is still under review. Deficiencies of this compound can result in convulsions, increased headaches, anemia, nausea, vomiting, dizziness, fatigue, hyperirritability, personality changes, learning difficulties, memory impairments, and possibly even hair loss and skin changes. There have been reports of the association of carpal tunnel syndrome being associated with deficiency of this compound. (Pizzorno, 2006)

Caution:

Prolonged use of vitamin B6 in rather large doses (1000 milligrams or greater per day) has been suggested to be toxic and may actually cause nerve damage or loss of coordination. As with any supplement, it is important to review its use with your physician or allied healthcare professional.

Folic Acid (Vitamin B-9)

Folic acid is also known as folacin. Folic acid is extremely important in proper brain function and the production of energy. It provides an important role in the synthesis of DNA as well as formation of red blood cells. Thus, this is a vital compound as one of the B-vitamins. It functions as a coenzyme for DNA and RNA synthesis, is important to maintain healthy cell division and reproduction, and is vitally important in the prevention of depression and anxiety, in avoidance of insomnia. It also aids in the prevention of birth defects, specifically neural tube defects. It additionally is felt to have an important role in the prevention of cardiovascular and neurovascular disorders. Folic acid is vitally important in the regulation of homocysteine levels. When there are adequate levels of folic acid, homocysteine is metabolized to benign components. With a lack of adequate folic acid levels, the concern is the development and predisposition of the breakdown of

> **The Doctor Says...**
>
> Folic acid is important in the prevention of depression and anxiety, in avoidance of insomnia, and also the prevention of birth defects...

the amino acid methionine, resulting in high levels of homocysteine associated with increased risk of atherosclerosis, plaque formation, stroke, and heart attack. Thus, it is important to have adequate amounts of folic acid, vitamin-B6, and vitamin-B12 in an effort that homocysteine be converted to non-harmful amino acids. There is controversy about the use of folic acid and B6 and B12 in an effort to lower homocysteine levels. Part of this issue is that in general, up to two-thirds of the population cannot properly absorb folic acid in the form that they are receiving it. Thus, they must be given the formulation in a methylfolate manner; hence, methyltetrahydrofolate is a bioavailable form that will actually cross the blood brain barrier into the spinal fluid and supply folic acid necessary for appropriate interactions and functions needed by the brain. However, not all people can produce adequate amounts necessary for proper brain function. Thus, the deficiencies of folic acid can occur from various sources from too low of a dietary intake, to blockage of absorption from oral contraceptive use, anticonvulsants, alcohol, or tobacco.

This methylfolate form can be obtained through various pharmaceutical grade preparations. Please review this with your physician or allied healthcare professional. (Balch, 2006)

Folic acid, in its natural form, is found in foods such as yeast, spinach, lentils, orange juice, beets and peas, soy foods, chicken, brown rice, eggs, and whole grains. (Balch, 2006)

Much like issues with other food sources, if you take in a supplement but cannot absorb it, the supplement does not do you very much good. For those people who are genetically predisposed and unable to ultimately provide adequate amounts of folate in the central nervous system (CNS) to help with the removal of homocysteine, they may be at greater risk of the development of atherosclerosis in the CNS (Brain), resulting in neurovascular damage. Much more research is necessary to understand this complicated situation. Better data analysis of individuals with regard to the intake of what form of folic acid they are receiving and what metabolites they are able to make is vital in understanding the data as it is today.

Folic acid goes by a variety of names such as vitamin-B9, folate, or pteroylglutamic acid (PGA). Thus, the various uses of these different names can be somewhat confusing. Again, I suggest that you start to read and familiarize yourself on this issue of this extremely important supplement to maintain proper brain and bodily functions. You are probably already familiar that folic acid is extremely important in pregnancy and should be utilized at least three months prior to consideration of becoming pregnant. Standard doses are usually recommended in 400 micrograms, but many physicians will often recommend higher dosing. I suggest you review this with your obstetrician if you are considering pregnancy in the near future. The key important issue is to avoid neural tube defect, spina bifida and anencephaly. It is also important for proper development of the brain and the body in general.

Keep in mind that on the various foods that are mentioned where folic acid can be consumed naturally, it is destroyed very easily by cooking; thus it is important that you do consume raw vegetables and fruits, as I discussed earlier, that can help you to maintain a proper balance of folic acid. Adequate amounts of folic acid have been felt to be important for facilitation of proper memory function and general healthy brain function. (Balch, 2006)

Vitamin B-12 (Cobalamin)

Vitamin B-12 is important for the proper function of the nervous system. It is needed to regulate the formation of red blood cells and to prevent anemia. Vitamin B-12 is required for the proper absorption and metabolism of carbohydrates and fats. It is linked to the production of acetylcholine, a vital neurotransmitter for proper memory function. Vitamin B -12 is also felt to aid in enhancing a good night sleep.

Vitamin B-12 comes in several forms. The form that is considered to be the most effective is methylcobalamin. The present, more common supplement form is cyanocobalamin, which is more difficult for our bodies to absorb. Intrinsic factor is a protein produced in your gastrointestinal tract and is needed for the proper absorption of Cobalamin (B-12). It is felt that bacteria in the intestines synthesize the majority of our vitamin B-12. (Balch, 2006)

Vitamin B-12 deficiency is common in the elderly and can be caused by malabsorption due to an absence of intrinsic factor. The deficiency can cause macrocytic anemia and neurological, psychiatric disorders. Younger individuals with gastric or intestinal disease can also develop these symptoms due to malabsorption. Individuals who suffer from depression and /or memory loss should have their B-12 level checked by their physician or allied healthcare professional.

Vitamin B-12 deficiency can also be associated with constipation, dizziness, headaches/migraines, inflammation of the tongue, moodiness, gait disorder, spinal cord degeneration, pernicious anemia, palpitations, and chronic fatigue.

Vegetarians (strict) will require vitamin B-12 supplementation because this vitamin is found almost exclusively in animal tissues. (Balch, 2006)

Individuals who are suffering from vitamin B-12 deficiency will need to get appropriate treatment from their physician or allied healthcare professional. Individuals who lack intrinsic factor or have a gastric or intestinal disorder will have to use a sublingual form, or preferably, the injection form of vitamin B-12 supplementation.

Vitamin B-12 is found in all meats, eggs, liver, fish (herring, mackerel), seafood, kidney, brewer's yeast, and milk. It is found in sea vegetables and soybeans, but not in other vegetables. Vitamin B-12 is also present in alfalfa and hops. (Balch, 2006)

Magnesium

Magnesium is involved in energy production and thus is vital to maintaining a healthy neuromuscular system. A deficiency in magnesium can result in abnormal transmissions of both muscle and nerve cells, resulting in a series of clinical symptoms that include sleep difficulties, irritability, rapid heartbeat, confusion, muscle cramps, GI upset, dizziness, depression, muscle twitching and possibly even convulsions in pregnant women. Proper magnesium is essential and important during pregnancy, but also throughout our entire life. Sources of magnesium can be found in: various dairy products, fish, meats, seafood, apples, apricots, avocados, bananas, grapefruits, nuts, sesame seeds and wheat. Proper supplementation is often needed and the chelated form is more easily absorbed and better tolerated by most individuals. (Pizzorno, 2006)

Chelated magnesium is recommended to begin at 200 milligrams daily and then increased as tolerated by 200 milligrams in 7 days to a target dose of 400 milligrams daily, or less as tolerated.

Vitamin C

The Doctor Says...
The body does not produce Vitamin C; it must be ingested as part of your diet.

Vitamin C is an essential antioxidant. It is required for hundreds of metabolic functions in the human body and is vital to your health. The body does not produce Vitamin C; it must be ingested as part of your diet. Vitamin C is vital in reducing the bad cholesterol, Low Density Lipoproteins (LDL) and helps to increase the good cholesterol, High Density Lipoproteins (HDL). It is vital in maintaining collagen, the integrity of your skin. It is helpful in avoiding blood clots and bruising, reducing the risk of cataracts, and promoting wound healing. ***For patients with memory loss it is vital to have both Vitamin C and E together*** to help to control free radical damage. This combination seems to be quite helpful on preserving cognitive function. (Pizzorno, 2006)

Caution for persons on anti-platelet or anticoagulation therapy:

Vitamin C, when taken with anti-platelet or anticoagulant therapies, can result in adverse events including: GI or intestinal ulcers and can interfere with the desired therapeutic function of the anti-platelet agents aspirin, clopidogrel, or [aspirin/dipyridamole], or the blood thinner agents, like warfarin. It is important that you review this issue with your healthcare professional. Should you be taking any medications to help prevent the neurovascular and/or cardiovascular diseases (stroke or heart attack), you should restrict yourself to a minimal amount of this vitamin supplement, since large amounts can result in adverse events or possible injury.

Vitamin D

Vitamin D is a prohormone that is necessary for the absorption and utilization of calcium and phosphorus. It is required for normal growth and maintenance of your bones, helps to regulate your heart rate, enhances immunity and is needed for normal blood clotting. (Balch, 2006)

Vitamin D has many forms: vitamin D2 (ergocalciferol) from food sources and vitamin D3 (cholecalciferol), synthesized in your skin after exposure to ultraviolet rays. The vitamin D3 (the natural form) is more effective than the vitamin D2 form. (Pizzorno, 2006)

The vitamin D that is found in food and in most supplements needs to be converted by the liver and kidney into the active form. Individuals with liver or kidney disorders are at increased risk of developing osteoporosis. In order to naturally get adequate amounts of vitamin D, you would need to ideally have 15 to 20 minutes exposure to sunlight at least three days per week. Ultraviolet sunlight exposure on the skin results in a cholesterol compound in the skin being transformed into the precursor of vitamin D, thus promoting the production. This becomes difficult for individuals living in northern regions during the winter. Vegetarians and the elderly may also be at risk of not getting an adequate amount of vitamin D. (Balch, 2006)

> **The Doctor Says...**
> In order to naturally get adequate amounts of vitamin D, you would need to ideally have 15 to 20 minutes exposure to sunlight at least three days per week.

Vitamin D is felt to have many other positive effects that may include: lowering coronary artery disease, reducing the risk of colon and breast cancer, and improving muscle strength, coordination, and strong bones.

Vitamin D deficiency can result in rickets in children and osteomalacia in adults. It can also be responsible for a loss of appetite, weight loss, insomnia, diarrhea, and visual difficulties. Vitamin D deficiency is more widespread in the elderly due to the potential decrease in exposure to sunlight, decreased intake of vitamin fortified foods, and deceased intestinal absorption. It must also be noted that the elderly produce about half the vitamin D after exposure to ultra-violet sunlight than younger adults. (Balch, 2006) (Pizzorno, 2006)

Vitamin D can be found in dairy products (milk, butter), fatty saltwater fish, tuna, salmon, halibut, sardines, oysters, cod liver oil, liver, oatmeal, fortified eggs, sweet potatoes, and vegetable oils. Some herbs also contain vitamin D: alfalfa and parsley. (Balch, 2006)

Liver, gallbladder and intestinal disorders can interfere with the proper absorption of vitamin D. Certain medications such as antacids, steroids, and cholesterol lowering drugs can block the absorption of vitamin D. If you are taking any of these medications, please review this issue with your physician or allied healthcare professional. (Balch, 2006)

Cautions:
     Toxicity can occur when individuals take excessive amounts of Vitamin D (>1000IU) (IU= International Units) daily, resulting in

decreased bone mass. It is recommended to take calcium along with vitamin D. (Balch, 2006)

Calcium

Calcium is vital in the proper maintenance of a fully functional healthy cardiovascular and neurovascular system. It is important in the regulation of our heart rate and vital in the importance of proper transmission in our nerve cells. It also has other very important roles with regard to the proper structure of our skeletal support system. It is vital in control of muscle contraction. Calcium is very important in cell membrane permeability and transmission throughout the entire body. Deficiencies in this compound can lead to a myriad of clinical symptoms such as joint pain, palpitations, hypertension, insomnia, muscle cramps, paresthesias, numbness, difficulty concentration, convulsions and depression. This is just a short list.

Calcium can be obtained in our diet in various natural sources such as skim milk, yogurt, cheeses, certain fish like salmon and sardines (which are also helpful in obtaining Omega 3 fish oil), broccoli, certain fruits (fortified orange juices, for example), in certain vegetables such as asparagus, and soybeans to name a few. (Bowden, 2007) There is a concern that calcium supplementation may actually interfere with individuals who have a history of kidney stones or kidney disease. There is question and controversy in this regard, but I suggest that this be reviewed with your physician or allied healthcare professional.

Calcium supplements have two components that can help promote a sound sleep; therefore, it may be beneficial to consider taking the compound in the evening. The normal range that people take is anywhere between 500 to 1500 milligrams a day. This compound is difficult to absorb in high quantities, so those doses exceeding 1000 milligrams may be difficult for the body to absorb. Thus, it would be suggested to take the product with meals spaced across the day and possibly at bedtime for the best possible absorption. You should take advantage of this attribute of calcium to help promote sleep. (Pizzorno, 2006)

Caution:

It must be noted that calcium is both influenced by the environment and can influence the environment, with regard to other medications. If you are taking various over-the-counter or prescription medications to control cardiac problems, palpitations, arrhythmias, abnormal heartbeat or for control of your blood pressure, you might be taking a medicine for which calcium in the supplement form may interfere with the proper function of the medicine, or vice versa. Should you be taking an anti-convulsant (anti-seizure medicine), some antibiotics such as tetracycline, or hormone supplementation such as thyroid, you may actually interfere with the absorption of the calcium and may not be getting the supplementation in the quantity that you desire or need clinically. If you are taking over-the-counter medicines on a regular basis, it is recommended you review with your physician or allied healthcare professional that you are taking this supplement since there can potentially be interference with the absorption of calcium and long-term problems if not addressed. Review any and all of these issues with your physician or allied healthcare professional. Calcium also cannot be taken with certain other compounds such as iron, because it will actually interfere with their absorption.

Vitamin E

Vitamin E is a complex compound. It is a powerful antioxidant with many subsets. Vitamin E is important in the prevention of cell damage by inhibiting the formation of free radicals. (Page, 2004) It helps protect the neurovascular and cardiovascular systems from the deleterious effects of low density lipoproteins (LDL), the bad cholesterol. It is also known to inhibit platelet aggregation. Thus, it inhibits potential clotting. For this reason, it is important to review the use of this product with your physician or allied healthcare professional, especially if you are taking an antiplatelet medication such as aspirin, clopidogrel [aspirin/dipyridamole], for example, where you may have a potential adverse event with the use of this compound depending on dosage and situation. Deficiencies of vitamin E may result in damage to the nervous system, impairment of neuromuscular function that interfere with the life span of the red blood cell and have several other potentially deleterious effects. Sometimes patients with difficulty with balance and coordination may actually have a deficiency of vitamin E and not be aware. It is

> **The Doctor Says...**
> Deficiencies of Vitamin E may result in damage to the nervous system.

important to obtain a high quality form of this compound, preferably the natural form of vitamin E. It is important to address the different subset families of this compound, noting that the d-alpha tocopherol acts as the antioxidant component. It is important to note that there are four subsets with regard to vitamin E the: alpha, beta, gamma and delta subsets. (Pizzorno, 2006) Vitamin E can be found in vegetables and in certain nuts   including soybean. It is found in corn, spinach, whole grains, whole wheat, and sunflower seeds, just to name a few. (Bowden, 2007)

Caution:

If vitamin E is taken in conjunction with anticoagulants (warfarin-blood thinner) or anti-platelet agents (aspirin, clopidogrel, [aspirin/dipyridamole]), consider using a lower dose range of 200 to 400 IU per day. Before starting vitamin E added supplementation, I strongly recommend that you review and monitor this with your physician or allied healthcare professional. Patients who are taking medications in the prevention of stroke or heart attack (or both) will need to address this key issue with regard to their supplement usage and their overall good health program. Periodic follow-ups with their physician or allied healthcare professional are an important part of general healthy brain program.

Coenzyme Q10 (CoQ10)

CoQ10 is essential in the production of adenosine triphosphate (ATP) which equals energy. It is critical for proper mitochondrial function. ATP is the immediate source of cellular energy in the human body. It is felt that a lack of sufficient coenzyme Q10 can lead to neurovascular and cardiovascular disease. Thus an adequate intake is essential on a daily basis (Balch, 2006).

In a placebo controlled study of CoQ10 in a dosage of 100mg given 3 times daily (TID) for 3 months, the CoQ10 proved to be significant in reducing migraine attack frequency. Dr. Rozen, in an open labeled study using CoQ10 150mg daily, demonstrated 61% of patients reported at least a 50% reduction in headache days per month. CoQ10 has been reported to be well tolerated with minimal side effects, even at higher doses. (Winner, 2008)

> **The Doctor Says...**
> CoQ10 proved to be significant in reducing migraine attack frequency.

Carnitine: Acetyl L Carnitine (ALC or ALCA)

Acetyl-L-Carnitine is a carnitine derivative that is produced by the body but often individuals are deficient. This is a very important compound in the efforts to control memory and to prevent the degeneration of the brain and nervous system. This compound has been studied and used in an effort to slow the progression of Alzheimer's dementia, to fight memory loss, and to help with attention and language function. It has also been considered for use in the treatment of depression.

Acetyl-L-Carnitine reportedly has other benefits: like enhancing the function of the immune system, and being a powerful antioxidant. It is primarily known for slowing cerebral aging and preserving and preventing nervous system disorders. It may also have a benefit in stress management with hormone regulation. The actual recommended daily dose of this compound ranges anywhere from 500 to about a thousand milligrams. At this time, there is no serious or toxic adverse event profile prominently known.

DHEA (Dehydroepiandrosterone)

DHEA (Dehydroepiandrosterone) is a hormone that is produced in the body. There are significant potential benefits with the use of this supplement, but it must be well respected. It is found naturally in the body, and associates with the hormones of testosterone, progesterone and corticosterone. It has been noted that DHEA declines with aging. The DHEA supplement has been utilized in an effort to assist in slowing the progression and prevention of memory disorder, to improve memory in the treatment of Alzheimer's dementia, and to be considered for other treatments such as lupus, osteoporosis and enhancing the immune system.

When this supplement is utilized, it is important to consider the addition of other antioxidants, such as Vitamin C and E, as well as the addition of Selenium in an effort to prevent some of the potential toxic effects on the liver. One of the ways to limit some of the potential side effects is to utilize the formulation of 7 Keto DHEA, which is not converted into estrogen or testosterone; thus, it has less of an adverse reaction. (Pizzorno, 2006)

There are potential benefits that have been studied with regard to DHEA, but there must be a judicious use of this compound. It is recommended that it be done under the supervision of your physician or allied healthcare professional, especially if it is to be utilized for any extended period of time.

.

Caution:

Caution needs to be exercised when taking this kind of a supplement, or any hormonal supplement. It is advisable to review the use of this medicine with your physician or allied healthcare professional before starting this supplement. While you are using this supplement, have periodic discussions and reviews with your healthcare professional as to whether or not any interventions need to be considered to monitor this hormone or the potentially influenced hormones such as testosterone or estrogen. Caution needs to be utilized when DHEA is considered in women with a history of breast cancer and men with a history of prostate cancer or enlarged prostate.

Ginkgo Biloba

Ginkgo Biloba has been utilized for hundreds, if not thousands of years, in an effort to improve memory function and to control muscle aches. It is an antioxidant and is felt to have anti-aging properties. It is normally well-tolerated and is often used in individuals that have a concern for memory loss and Alzheimer's. (Ulbricht, 2005)

> **The Doctor Says...**
> Ginkgo Biloba has been utilized for hundreds, if not thousands of years.

Glucosamine Sulfate

Glucosamine sulfate is a compound that contains an amino acid, glutamine, and a sugar, glucose, component. It is found in high concentrations in the human joint structures. It is found to have various helpful aspects as it relates to pain. It also may help to reduce the destruction of cartilage when patients are using other pain medicines such as non steroidals. You will sometimes see this compound combined with other compounds such as MSM, methylsulfonylmenthane. (Balch, 2006)

Caution:

If someone is allergic to sulfur they should not take this or any other sulfur compound.

MSM (Methylsulfonylmenthane)

MSM (Methylsulfonylmenthane) is a naturally occurring sulfur compound. This compound is felt to assist in controlling muscle pain. It also has benefit in headache and migraine, arthritic conditions and helps in the healing process of injuries, decreasing inflammation or relieving pain and possibly even helping in the GI system. The compound is often taken in the range from 1000 to 2000 milligrams. (Pizzorno, 2006)

Caution:

If someone is allergic to sulfur they should not take this or any other sulfur compound.

DLPA (DL- Phenylalanine)

> **The Doctor Says...**
> A combination of the DL may prove overall more beneficial for the control of general health or pain.

Phenylalanine has various formulations: the L, D and a DL form of this compound. This is one of the essential amino acids, which is vital in the synthesis of dopamine and norepinephrine, important neurotransmitters for proper maintenance of the central nervous system and proper brain health. They are involved in mood and pain control, memory, learning, and also may influence aspects with regard to weight management and proper BMI. They also may have even more far reaching aspects, since these are such vital neurotransmitters for proper brain function. The D form is known to be primarily effective in control of pain; the L form may also have control and assistance in this area, and it is felt to also assist with alertness and possible control of weight. A combination of the DL may prove overall more beneficial for the control of general health or pain. (Pizzorno, 2006)

This is a supplement that is recommended for short-term use during acute pain exacerbations. This is where it would have its best potential.

Caution:

This supplement should not be taken by pregnant women or patients who are suffering from diabetes, hypertension, who have a history of melanoma (skin cancer), concerns with regard to anxiety, panic attack or generalized anxiety disorder or social anxiety disorder, and patients who have difficulty with the metabolism of phenylalanine (PKU –phenylketonura). Should there be any concern about whether this supplement should be taken, review this with your physician or allied healthcare professional before beginning this compound. It is for short-term use for primarily acute pain.

Butterbur (Petasites hybridus)

Butterbur is a perennial found in Europe. The root of this potentially toxic plant needs to have the toxic pyrrolizidine alkaloids removed. (Skidmore-Roth, 2006)

It is felt to inhibit leukotriene synthesis, thus having a migraine neurogenic anti-inflammatory effect. Dr. Lipton demonstrated, in a randomized placebo controlled study, that 75mg of the extracted purified butterbur product given two times a day (BID) was statistically superior to placebo in the reduction of migraine frequency. It was reported to be well tolerated with minimal side effects reported except for burping. (Winner, 2008)

Caution:

Butterbur should be avoided during pregnancy and lactation. The pyrrolizidine alkaloids in this herb can cause irreversible hepatic damage.

Huperzine

Huperzine is felt to be potentially effective for increasing memory retention, alertness, language ability, and to help facilitate memory in patients with Alzheimer's dementia. It works by blocking acetylcholinesterase, the enzyme that is important in the activation of acetylcholine, thus leading to the importance of memory function.

This is a Chinese herb huperzina serrata. It is suggestive to utilize dosages of 50-75 mcg daily, in an effort to assist in this aspect. There is information with regard to much higher doses of this compound being used. As much as 200 mcg twice a day may be used to improve memory function in Alzheimer's patients. There have been no significant side effects generally noted with this compound.

(Pizzorno, 2006) Presently, clinical research is underway to address the potential effect of huperzine on memory function in patients with Alzheimer's.

CAUTION:

If the person is already taking an acetylcholinesterase inhibitor, there is potential toxicity should this compound be used in conjunction. Please review with your physician or allied healthcare professional since huperzine is a potentially potent inhibitor of acetylcholinesterase, and you would be taking two compounds doing relatively similar functions. The potential for toxicity of this combination is clearly a concern.

Vinpocetine

Vinpocetine is an extract of periwinkle, a derivative of vincamine. It has been felt to help enhance memory by improving blood flow to the CNS and improving ATP, oxygen and glucose utilization. It is felt to also guard against stroke and possibly have some beneficial effects against balance and hearing loss. Further study is clearly needed with regard to this compound. The dosing is suggested to be anywhere from 5-10 mg daily. (Pizzorno, 2006)

Phosphatidyl Serrine

Phosphatidyl Serrine is purified from lecithin concentrate. This compound is felt to help play a role in improving nerve cell function and conduction. It crosses the blood-brain barrier and is felt to help in improving cognitive ability, memory, and learning, especially in patients with memory disorder such as Alzheimer's. This compound can be found and often derived through soybeans. Doses of 40-100 mg are suggested.

The clinical benefits of this compound seem to be more apparent in brain related functions, cognition, mood, and stress management with regard to these phospholipid compound. This compound is felt to help optimize brain function. This compound seems to possibly diminish the symptoms of mood disorder in depressed individuals; thus, it may add to its beneficial effect on memory and cognition. Benefits come from the clear link with depression and impaired memory, especially in older people. This compound does not seem to have a direct affect on the levels of serotonin, thus it suggests a different mechanism of action with regard to its control of depression and memory. (Pizzorno, 2006)

Although the dosing tends to be roughly about 100 mg daily, this compound has been used in higher doses of up to 300-500 mg daily. Further research is needed with regard to this compound.

CAUTION:

No adverse events or interactions have been noted with this compound, although it must be noted that upset stomach has been reported in some individuals taking this compound.

Bocopa

Bocopa monniera is an Ayurvedic botanical compound that is felt to help enhance memory, diminish insomnia, and may prove to have mild sedative qualities. It is felt to be most beneficial to prevent memory dysfunction. It is felt that this compound works by diminishing DNA damage from free radical formation. The dosage of this compound is suggested to be roughly about 80 mg daily. Further study is needed regarding this compound and its use in memory disorders. (Pizzorno, 2006)

Summary

The first part of this chapter discussed an overview of the supplements that you should be taking as they may be considered in the management of Healthy Brain Wellness, Migraine/Headache, Memory Loss, Pain, Stroke, and Sleep. These are supplements that you should consider taking on a daily basis to keep your brain functioning at full capacity. The respective sections give you specific directions on how to most effectively use supplements and improve your brain and bodily function. The second part of the chapter comprehensively reviewed the effects of each individual supplement. This section is for more detailed information, and to be used as a reference.

References and Recommended Reading

Balch PA. Prescription for Nutritional Healing. 4th ed. New York, NY: Avery Penguin Group; 2006.pp3-807.

Basch EM, Ulbricht CE. Natural Standard Herb & Supplement Handbook. St. Louis, Missouri: Elsevier Mosby; 2005. pp 25-937.

Bowden J. The 150 Healthiest Foods on Earth. Gloucester, Mass: Fair Winds Press; 2007. pp 8-324.

Breus M. Good Night. New York, NY: Dutton; 2006. pp1-283.

Chopra D. Alternative Medicine. 2nd ed. Berkeley, CA: Celestial Arts; 2002. pp557-938.

Hobbs C, Haas E. Vitamins for Dummies. Hoboken, NJ: Wiley Publishing, Inc.;1999.pp1-318.

Logan AC. The Brain Diet. Nashville, Tennessee: Cumberland House; 2006, 2007. pp1-277.

Null G. The Complete Encyclopedia of Natural Healing. New York, NY: Kensington Books; 1998. pp3-712.

Page L. Healthy Healing 12th ed. Healthy Healing, Inc.; 2004. pp289-623.

Pizzorno JE, Murray M. Textbook of Natural Medicine. 3rd ed. St. Louis, Missouri: Churchill Livingstone Elsevier; 2006. pp 709-2201.

Roizen MF,Oz MC. You on a Diet. New York, NY: Free Press; 2006. pp3-354.

Silberstein SD, Lipton RB, Dodick DW. Wolff's Headache. New York, NY: Oxford University Press; 2008. pp3-824.

Skidmore-Roth L. Mosby's Handbook of Herbs & Natural Supplements 3rd ed. St. Louis, Missouri: Elsevier Mosby; 2006. pp1-923.

Tribole E. The Ultimate Omega-3 Diet. New York, NY: McGraw Hill: 2007. pp1-324.

Ulbricht CE, Basch EM. Natural Standard Herb & Supplement Reference. St. Louis, Missouri: Elsevier Mosby; 2005. pp 22-789.

Victor M, Ropper AH. Adams and Victor's Principles of Neurology. 7th ed. New York: McGraw -Hill Medical Publishing Division; 2001pp45-1644.

Winner P, Lewis DW, Rothner AD. Headache in Children and
    Adolescents 2nd ed. Hamilton, Ontario: BC
    Decker, Inc.; 2008 pp1-314.

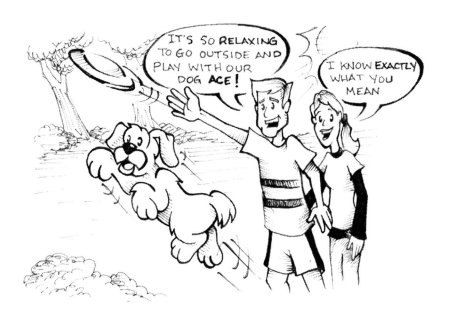

Step 3: Stress Management

      "Learn to manage stress, or stress will manage you!" One of my professors once said "...we all need a little stress in our life; otherwise we will not function at our highest levels of efficiency". The key is to recognize the level of stress that is helpful and the level that is harmful. Use this knowledge to manage your ideal stress level throughout your life.

      Stress is definitely one of the main causes of many chronic illnesses that we see in the field of neurology and, indeed, all fields of medicine. For example, stress can

> **The Doctor Says...**
> Stress can certainly precipitate migraine headaches.

certainly precipitate migraine headaches. It also increases the risk of a whole host of other conditions: heart disease, hypertension, gastrointestinal problems, reflux, irritable bowel, depression and body weight issues. In this chapter, we will address issues on how to recognize stress and give you suggestions on how to deal with it. You need to manage your stress, so that your stress does not manage you.

Stress comes in many different forms. Our environment is one source; bad weather, pollen, pollution, noise, traffic are daily components of life for most of us. Socially, we must deal with our families, friends, co-workers, bosses, teachers and schoolmates. We face daily, ongoing challenges at work and school. Medical issues, illness and injury can often be overwhelming physically, psychologically, and financially. Sometimes, stressors are all consuming, and our thinking becomes clouded. This is often when we make poor diet choices, do not sleep well, and try to alleviate the pressure with alcohol or medication. We end up creating a situation where we do not take care of ourselves, thereby making these situations worse. Remember, taking care of yourself should be a top priority.

> **The Doctor Says...**
> Taking care of yourself should be a top priority.

Forms of Stress

There are two key forms of stress: Acute and Chronic.

Acute stress is a protective mechanism, otherwise known as our "fight or flight" response. This mechanism is what we use when there is immediate and possibly life-threatening danger present. This response serves us well, for instance, if there is about to be an accident. Our senses are sharpened and our reflexes and responses are heightened. This mechanism happens because our bodies release norepinephrine, more commonly known as adrenaline, which increases our heart and breathing rates, speeds up metabolism, and raises blood pressure. Your muscles tense, your pupils dilate and your hearing becomes more acute. You are ready to take on the danger or to flee as fast as you can. This response has served us well throughout our evolution.

What happens if our fight or flight response is subjected to chronic stress, unchecked perception of danger, or exposure to a perceived threat for a long period of time? Such norepinephrine overload can inhibit proper brain function and adversely affect many organs. Our immune system response is diminished and inflammatory responses increase, all of which are deleterious to our ultimate health and well-being. Fortunately, the body can turn off the fight or flight response as quickly as it can turn it on. We call this a relaxation response. (Winner, J. 2003) After the perceived threat is no longer a concern, your brain will begin the process through the nervous system

of shutting down the fight or flight response. Your heart rate,
breathing, and blood pressure will return to normal levels. Dr. Herbert Benson in 1975 coined the term, "The Relaxation Response", noting that we have the ability to help improve our own personal health by

The Doctor Says...
We have the ability to help improve our own personal health by learning to relax.

learning to relax. This control ultimately prevents inappropriate fight
or flight responses. (Winner,J. 2003) I will address relaxation
techniques in more detail later in the chapter.

The second form of stress is chronic stress. Chronic stress
comes in many forms. Some people see their jobs as a source of
chronic stress. They think of a long protracted work load, the burden
of quotas, or the possibility of losing their position. Sometimes
chronic stress results from personal issues such as a divorce, the loss
of several loved ones, or a potentially life-threatening illness such as
cancer. As long as you perceive a significant threat for a prolonged
period of time you are clearly at risk from the effects of chronic stress.

We know that chronic stress can lead to persistent muscle
discomfort, tension, fatigue, hypertension, migraines, and
gastrointestinal issues like ulcers. Pulmonary conditions such as
asthma or bronchitis worsen with stress. Unhealthy weight
fluctuations, particularly weight gain, can lead to conditions such as
diabetes. Chronic stress can also interfere in our personal relationships
in many ways; loss of libido is a common side effect. And because

stress can exacerbate our inflammatory systems, the aging process is significantly quickened.

Today, many medical practices, including mine, are now addressing the issues of chronic stress, disease, aging and their interrelationship to progressive neurologic disorders. Stress is often a factor in many illnesses, as well as a disease in and of itself. This disease must be addressed, diagnosed, and treated. The key to addressing chronic stress is not eradication, but management. We can change our attitude toward stress and learn to use it as a stepping stone towards personal growth.

There have been various studies addressing both good and bad stress. There are many excellent stress management workbooks available today. I suggest that you consider working through some of these. One that you may find very helpful is called "Relaxation and Stress Reduction Workbook", presently in its fifth edition by authors Martha Davis, PhD., Elizabeth Robins Eshelman M.S.W., and Matthew McKay, PhD. It is important to recognize the various stresses that we are exposed to over the course of a one to two year period. At times we can handle these stresses on our own, but at other times we will need to seek professional assistance from physicians or allied healthcare professionals.

We need to look at stress as a challenge, an opportunity to improve our own personal self. We need to look at it in the most positive light, learn to work through it in a constructive way, and prevent it from having a deleterious effect on our lives.

Throughout the rest of this chapter we are going to break down the aspects of stress so we can better understand it and discuss coping techniques. Simple things such as appropriate exercise, proper foods, proper balance of antioxidants, learning to balance our personal, social, and business calendars, keeping an optimistic attitude and learning to laugh out loud every day are keys to successfully managing stress.

Relaxation

Just as change is synonymous with stress, meditation is synonymous with the relaxation response. Meditation is simply a relaxation technique. Learning methods of meditation will ultimately lead to far less stress and a much more enjoyable lifestyle.

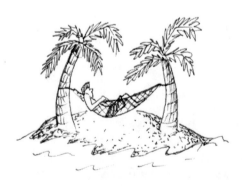
A simple way of learning meditation is to learn diaphragmatic breathing. This method of breathing requires you to breathe in through your nose and let your diaphragm move upward, resulting in your abdomen contracting. There are several ways to perform this exercise. Try several and find the one that works best

for you. A simple way is to breathe in slowly through the nose for a count of five and feel your abdomen going in as your diaphragm goes up. Hold your breath for a count of five and then slowly exhale through your mouth for a count of five. Repeat this exercise several times and you will find that you begin to relax. (Winner,J. 2003) If you have never done this before, it may take a few times before you become comfortable with diaphragmatic breathing. There is an excellent book written by Jay Winner, M.D. called "Stress Management Made Easy", which can make learning relaxation techniques much easier. This book also has CDs that accompany the text. It is important to become comfortable with some form of meditation, and diaphragmatic breathing is one of the simplest and easiest methods. You can do it anywhere, anytime, under any circumstance.

> **The Doctor Says...**
> Sometimes even just a simple deep breath in a stressful situation is all that is necessary to curb stress.

Sometimes even just a simple deep breath in a stressful situation is all that is necessary to curb stress.

It is important to find enjoyable, healthy physical activities that you can do on a routine basis. Walking, hiking, biking, and swimming are all activities requiring little or no equipment. Vary the routine and try to do some form of exercise three to five times a week for at least 30 minutes. You need to fit this in despite your busy schedule. Often, it is easier to find time for exercise first thing in the morning. When this is

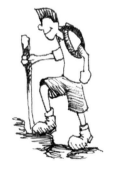

not possible, try to schedule one of the activities in the early part of the evening, preferably just after work. It is advisable not to do any strenuous exercises 2-3 hours before sleep because it may interfere with your proper sleep patterns. More on sleep and proper preparation for sleep will be addressed in a later chapter of this book.

Another technique of stress management is to find something you really look forward to and try to include it in your daily routine. It could be just a simple walk with your dog, spending time with your pet, listening to music, calling a friend to put a smile on your face, or even visiting a website that has jokes to make you laugh.

Attitude

Our attitude is key to the management of stress. We can choose to react to a situation and increase our own stress by seeing the negative and being fearful, or we can choose a more positive approach

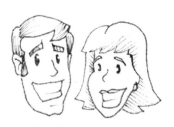

and look for the good. We can come to realize that we are in control of our responses to the events in our life. We often feel that the outside environment controls us, and that our emotions result from the uncontrollable circumstances that surround us. This is just not true; these are the times when we most need to take control and use the many stress reduction tools that are easy to learn and implement.

It is important to get in the habit of focusing. In times of stress, revert back to breathing from your diaphragm. Do not take shallow quick breaths when you are under pressure; take deep breaths using your diaphragm. Try to focus on a pleasant thought or memory. When possible, make your surroundings peaceful and comfortable. Hang a picture on the wall that makes you smile. Use aroma therapies. Surround yourself with music that gives you a tranquil feeling.

Enjoy the moment! Try not to live in the past or worry about the future. Watch the sunset. Enjoy that beautiful afternoon on your walk to or from work. Notice a blue jay sitting on a branch as you walk into work in the morning. Enjoy walking your dog in the morning, even though it might make you a few minutes late for work. Life is a gift, remember to say thank you!

Stress can be a positive force. Oftentimes when we have a project deadline, for example, stress creates energy that can be channeled and used creatively. Set goals that you feel you can achieve. Even when you feel you've "bitten off more than you can chew", enjoy the learning process instead of worrying about what you cannot do. It has been said that the journey is often more exciting than the destination.

We are less stressed when we can focus on one goal or project at a time. It seems our society relishes the idea of multi-tasking. As human beings, we are far more efficient and far less stressed when we uni-task. I suggest that you learn to focus and complete one task at a time when at all possible. Help spread these concepts to your coworkers, friends, and family: everyone benefits!

Control Your Own Thoughts

There are all kinds of discussions about internal and external centers of control. ***The reality is you control your own destiny; you control your responses, your attitude and your behavior.*** You choose the goals you wish to achieve. You choose to accept a failure as a failure or as nothing more than an outcome that needs to be fixed. After all, failure is a great opportunity to learn from your mistakes. ***The key to the equation is you.*** Sir Winston Churchill once said "Success is the ability to go from one failure to another with no loss of enthusiasm". He also said, "The pessimist sees difficulty in every opportunity; the optimist sees opportunity in every difficulty".

The key to addressing this locus of control is to realize that the externals are not the key to happiness. We control our response to a stressful situation, our ability to obtain satisfaction and make the choices ourselves that lead to our own calm response. Thus, it is key to develop your internal locus of control if you wish to manage stress in your life successfully. There is a wonderful book that speaks to this point by W. Mitchell called "It's Not What Happens To You, It's What You DO About It" that wonderfully illustrates the importance of an internal locus of control when dealing with stress. (Winner, J. 2003)

Your Personality

Lighten up! Learn to accept yourself. Learn to be kind to yourself and do not be so hard on yourself when you fail or do not achieve a goal in your set timeline. Learn to forgive yourself.

Whether you are a type "A" or a type "B" personality, accept yourself for who you are. Both personalities have plus and minus aspects. Emphasize the positive and deemphasize the negative of your personality. We have all been given gifts; we need to recognize them. We have all been given talents; we need to use them. Some of us are lucky enough to recognize these gifts and talents at a very early age, and have been surrounded by people who encourage and nurture us. We are not all that fortunate. However, we do have a lifetime to discover these talents and use them.

> **The Doctor Says...**
> We have all been given gifts; we need to recognize them.

In our fast-paced world we often go from one task or goal to another, unmindful of the time rushing by. There is an old saying, "take time to smell the roses". Truer words have never been spoken.

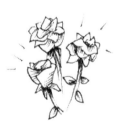

It is important to integrate relaxation into your life. Recognize your personality and find what fits best for you.

Whatever your personality type, try to spend a little more time with your friends and your family. Make a weekly call to a brother, sister, mother, father, or grandparent who does not live in your area and just say hello; you will both feel better for it. Call a close friend daily. Statistics show that a strong network of friends is a guaranteed stress reducer. Become a better listener; try not to interrupt people when they speak. Try this exercise: pick the longest line in a department store or grocery store and enjoy the wait. Watch the people around you. Watch the environment. Watch the interactions. Wait long enough and you will surely see something very comical! You will probably also see someone you actually can help. Either way you will leave with a smile on your face. Take an hour out of the day and do absolutely nothing. Can you do it? Many of us would find it impossible!

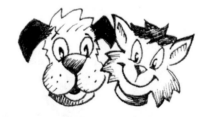

If you do not have a pet, consider getting one. Pet therapy is clearly helpful to all people. It has been successful in nursing homes and hospitals. Why not enjoy these benefits in your own home?

Cultivate a hobby, something you really look forward to doing. Get involved in cultural activities, museums, art shows, concerts, and opera. Find something you like and do it often. **Remember to include "fun stuff" on your To Do List**, not just all chores.

If you find yourself under a lot of stress, take your To Do List and remove 25% of the items immediately, then look at the 75% that are left and pick the top 1-3 that absolutely must be done that day. Do your best to accomplish those and do not worry about anything else on 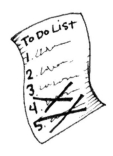 that list. Do this every day and you should feel less stressed.

Another way to control stress is to look at your emails once a day. Now, this may not be possible in every person's job, but try. In the beginning, if you are looking at your email constantly all day long, try to limit it to a few minutes at lunchtime and at the end of your work day. Gradually, over the course of 2-4 weeks go to them once a day. (Ferriss T. 2007) Constantly looking at email is unproductive and ultimately will lead to more stress. Obviously there are exceptions. Some jobs require constant email interaction. For those of us who do not require such diligence, you will find this an amazingly simple approach to decreasing your stress.

Thank You

Be thankful every day for what you have. Remember to say thank you every time someone helps you. ***There is a miracle in being grateful, and there is enormous power in saying thank you.*** Be grateful for the little and the big things in your life. Count your blessings every day.   One of the foundations for a positive attitude and for powerful stress management is learning to be grateful, learning to say thank you, and learning to be appreciative. I must admit that I am not always the best at this and I work hard every day now to tell the people in my life how much I appreciate them. If you are married, it starts with your spouse and kids. If you are fortunate enough to have your parents or grandparents, include them. Remember your fellow students and coworkers. None of us can accomplish our goals without help. There are many people we never see and never meet whom ultimately lead to our success every day. People that help deliver food to the grocery stores and make sure that we have electricity and clean water certainly deserve our thanks. Teachers, medical personnel, police and fire fighters… the list goes on and on.

Every day we have beautiful things that surround us all the time: a sunrise, a rainbow, a rain shower, a thunderstorm, the companionship of a friend, family members, greeting from a pet, the challenges given to us at work and school, and the opportunities given to us at work and school.

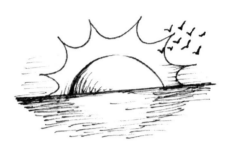

I advise you to participate in volunteer work with people less fortunate than yourself. When you help someone that is less fortunate, you help yourself and you often learn to recognize how fortunate you are. You will begin the process of truly being grateful for the gifts and talents you have. You also sometimes find and develop talents you did not even realize you had. Either way you ultimately control your own stress and improve the quality of your own life while you are helping someone else. This is a win-win situation! Keep in mind that when we help people with their problems, we spend less time focusing on ours. Sometimes our problems seem far more insignificant compared to those of the people we help. What a great way to put things into perspective.

Laugh Out Loud

It is important to laugh everyday early and often. If there is someone funny

> **The Doctor Says...**
> It is important to laugh everyday, early and often.

at work or in school, stay around them as much as you can, for the more you smile, the less stress you have, the longer you will live, and the better quality of life you will experience. Today, the internet has a lot of funny places to get jokes. You can even have them sent to you daily. If you find a funny website that makes you laugh, visit it every day for a few minutes. Make it part of your own laugh therapy. If you are fortunate enough to be one of those talented people that can make people laugh, go ahead and have fun. Now we do have to be careful in the topics we choose these days, but there are plenty of ways to make people laugh while staying within appropriate social moralities.

Today

Remember, we only have today. It does not pay to dwell on the past. Tomorrow is something we can look forward to, but not something we should worry about or fear. Make the best of everyday; keep enjoying every moment you possibly can. Should you be put into a significantly stressful situation, try to use your meditation techniques. We have discussed the simplest of these: take deep breaths until you begin to relax. Focus on a pleasant memory or go to a place where you are comfortable and can relax, either at home, work, or just in your mind. We do have a limited time on this planet. We need to be mindful of that, thus we need to enjoy every day that we have.

There is a very interesting book that can help us with perspectives of stress management. It's called "Don't Sweat the Small Stuff", and I highly recommend that you read this book. It will make you reflect on specific aspects of life and you will surely laugh at certain chapters. There are several versions of this book that have been published, but I suggest that you begin with the original version: "Don't Sweat the Small Stuff, It's All Small Stuff" by Richard Carlson.

How Much is Enough?

How many things do we need to own? How many material things will really make us happy? It's not the cars, the houses, the electronic equipment, or the video games that will ultimately give us peace, balance and help us to manage our stress at the end of the day. Clearly, these items will give us some joy for a few moments and they can be used appropriately as part of stress management, but they are not really the final answer. We should not be preoccupied with money and possessions. Once we meet the basic needs for ourselves and our families, we need to focus on helping others. A large portion of our well being is centered on family, friends, and a sense of community. True wealth is having a loving family and devoted and loving friends. The true measure of success is this: Did you leave this world a better place than you found it? Have you put a smile on a child's face? Have you given a helping hand to a stranger? Has one person's life been improved because of you? If you have answered yes to any of these questions, you are a success. That is often all it takes to reduce the stress in your life.

Balance

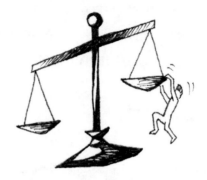

Achieving a successful balance between family and career is really a key component in stress management. Finding the right balance is easier said than done! Let's look at some helpful hints and some suggested reading that will help you achieve this goal.

Full Speed Ahead

Many of us work at one-hundred miles an hour, 100% of the time. We do not give ourselves any margin for error. It's no wonder we are stressed out. Go back to the 25% suggestion: look at your day and remove at least 25% of the items on your To Do List. Give yourself a margin of error. Allow for mishaps. Allow for traffic. Allow for problems getting on the computer. Allow for something unexpected to occur during the day. This alone will help reduce your stress each day. It is okay if your inbox does not get emptied every day. The key is to learn to focus on the most important items that need to be done that day and do them first. Again, easier said than done, but if we work at it, it will become a habit with rich rewards! Look at the remaining items with a positive attitude. Find ways to enjoy them. Perhaps recruiting a friend or co-worker to assist you might lighten the burden. Delegation is a great way to increase efficiency. It can also be a mentoring process for someone who may be eager to learn new skills.

Remember to give yourself and your co-workers a little bit of slack and forgiveness. This activity is a great chance for you to use your talents to help someone else. You have reduced your workload for the day, you have actually gotten someone else involved, you helped teach that individual, and ultimately, they will be a great asset. They are now more appreciative, and the increased responsibility boosts their self-esteem. Most people want to help someone else. Most people take enormous joy in being needed, the elderly included. Many times people retire and are "put out to pasture". These people have a lot to offer. Get them involved in your life. They may turn out to be some of your best friends and give you some of the most important wisdom on the planet. Do not forget our elderly, they offer us valuable life experiences.

Exercise

We are going to address this topic in great detail in another chapter of this book, but exercise is important in stress management. Make it part of your daily routine; it is easier than you think. Instead of finding the parking spot closest to the store, look for the spot that is furthest away. Enjoy the scenery on the way, enjoy a shop window, and engage in some people-watching. Because you took the longer path, you may meet an old friend you have not seen for months. This is a great way to spend your lunch hour, or a wonderful de-stressor at the end of your day. Exercise comes in many forms, not just on the treadmill. Make a real effort to include exercise as part of your normal routine during your week. It is important to exercise at least 30 minutes several times a week, preferably every day. Dr. Michael Roizen and Dr. Mehmet Oz, in their book "You on a Diet", place great importance on exercise and suggest that you should at least walk everyday for 20-30 minutes. I refer you to that book if you have not

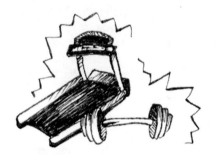

already read it. It is an excellent text addressing diet and has many suggestions for exercise as well as managing stress. Before embarking on any exercise program or changing any dietary or supplement program, it is important that you review these issues with your physician or allied healthcare professional, especially if you have an existing medical condition.

Avoid the Excesses

It is important to understand that there are certain items that may seem to help us in the short run in controlling our stress, but in the long run can be detrimental. Using illicit drugs to control stress will end up creating problems that will result in far more serious physical and psychological problems.

There are some subtle issues. Caffeine is actually useful, and most people enjoy a cup or two daily. If you are consuming large quantities, however, you may want to review this issue with your physician or allied healthcare professional. Clearly, if you are trying to use this to get through the day, there may be some underlying medical condition that may have to be worked up and addressed.

Alcohol is often used by people to control stress and again there are some discussions about the benefit of small doses of alcohol and the benefits of some ingredients in wine. The key is to review this issue with your physician or allied healthcare professional, along with the potential benefits or risks depending on your medical condition. Enjoying a glass of wine with dinner 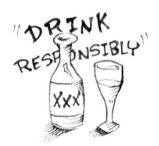 is one thing; using alcohol to excess can cause very serious health problems. Again, speak to your doctor or healthcare professional about healthier stress control alternatives.

Stress Foods

In the section on nutrition, we address more detailed information on healthy foods that can be utilized to improve your quality of life and ultimately help you manage stress. When it comes to your healthy diet and managing stress, it is important to review some basics. Do not skip breakfast, and choose appropriate foods. Avoid significantly high caloric intakes of foods that are low in nutrient content, high in sugar content, and high in trans fats and saturated fats that can ultimately lead to obesity or insulin resistance and potentially diabetes. Avoid excessive consumption of carbonated soft drinks. This is not the way to control our stress and it is surely not the way to have a healthy diet, develop a healthy brain, a healthy body, and a healthy lifestyle. A routine that we do every day is eating. Focus on healthy foods. It is important as a part of stress management to have a good high quality breakfast. Look forward to that. Set up breakfast meals that you enjoy, ultimately leading to reduction of your stress. What does that mean? Avoid high sugar, low fiber type breakfasts. That doughnut tastes great, but ultimately it is not great for us.

Some examples of a good breakfast are a nice bowl of fruit such as blueberries, raspberries, and strawberries mixed with a banana 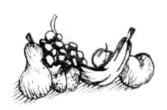 (not too ripe) or pears, peaches, and plums. Vary these fruits. Pick fruits that you really like, but try to avoid too much intake of grapes and overripe fruit. Other options for breakfast: two or three eggs, preferably the Omega-3 enriched eggs (please refer to the nutritional section of this book for more details). A high fiber, high quality cereal with skim milk is also a good choice. Many supplements can be taken in the morning with a good breakfast. Vary your breakfast routine so you will look forward to eating in the morning. Now that you have started your day with a healthy breakfast and appropriate supplements, you are on the fast track to beating stress!

If you find that you must eat something during stressful moments, try fruit. Keep an apple, pear, peach, banana, or a plum close by. Have a drink of water. Try green tea or some other herbal tea that you enjoy. Avoid reaching for that piece of pastry or caffeinated carbonated beverage.

Pseudo Stress Buster

Sometimes we feel we are overweight. There is a really simple way to address this. Calculate your BMI. If the result is 25 or over, then numerically you are overweight. A BMI of 30 or over puts you in the obese category and it is appropriate to get in contact with your doctor or healthcare professional and design a suitable regime to lose that weight. Weight control is important for brain and heart health. Going on a diet can be a stressful event, but learning about the long term benefits of weight loss makes the effort worthwhile.

Stress Diet

The first issue is to decide how much weight you want to lose. Understand that as soon as you decide to go on a diet, you are entering into a stressful situation for your mind and your body. For example, if you decide that you are going to lose 20 pounds, you must set a goal and a timeline that are reasonable. Twenty pounds may be fine if that is what it takes for you to achieve a normal BMI (between 18 and 24.9).   Remember to give yourself adequate time to lose anything more than a few pounds. It can take months to properly lose 20 pounds. The key is not just losing the pounds, it is maintaining the loss. There are several efficient ways to lose weight. I would suggest, again, that you review any significant weight loss program in great detail with your physician or allied healthcare professional before starting. Make sure you are healthy enough to do this, and make sure you pick a diet regime that is best for you. See Figure 4.

Figure 4

Keep in Mind Some Simple Dietary Aspects:

1) Choose good quality food at all times
2) Understand it is okay to be a little hungry
3) Try not to eat by the clock, but eat small portions of well balanced foods when you are hungry

Understand that foods eaten in the morning may be used by your body in a different way than when the same food is eaten at night or in combination with other foods. For example, fruit is often best utilized when taken early in the meal such as part of breakfast or as an appetizer during lunch or dinner. Portion size is important, and you need to eat enough fruits and vegetables throughout the day. We do need a little fat in our diet each day, but we need the right kind of fats. Fish and eggs rich in Omega-3 and the fats in olive oil are good examples of the "right kind" of fat. These are just some suggestions. Again I refer you to several excellent books on the issue of diet and nutrition as it relates to heart and brain health. My suggestions are "You on a Diet" by Dr. Michael Roizen and Dr. Mehmet Oz; "The Ultimate Omega-3 Diet by Evelyn Trobole, M.S.; "The Reality Diet" by Dr. Steven Schnur; "The Best Life Diet" by Bob Greene; and "The Brain Diet" by Alan Logan, N.D. I suggest you also review other established dietary programs. The key is to do your research and educate yourself on these issues. Eat when you are hungry, but stop eating before you are full. It can take 30 to 45 minutes for the brain to get the message that there is enough food in the stomach, so it is important to eat slowly. In our society, we tend to have a 5-15 minute lunch break because we have so many things besides eating to be done during our lunch hour. It goes back to the one-hundred miles an hour for 100% of the time concept. For your lunch break, have lunch and nothing else. I know this is not always practical but it is worth trying!

The Power of Family and Friends

Do not underestimate the power of your personal social support system. Your immediate family, your extended family, your close friends, and even your colleagues at work all make up your social support system. Those of us who have a strong social support system have a lot less stress in our lives. We have other people with whom we can share our problems and concerns. They share the joy of our successes and the pain of our defeats. We take joy in making them happy as well. We all have experienced the fun of looking for a gift for family or a special friend. Giving is truly more fun than receiving!

Communication

> **The Doctor Says...**
> The key to communication is listening, not speaking.

The key to communication is listening, not speaking. Often we are so concerned about getting our point across that we do not hear a word the other person is saying. Sit back one day and just observe conversations amongst your friends, family or coworkers. Pay attention to how people listen. Notice how few people actually listen to the other person. Try this exercise: when you are in a conversation with someone wait until they are completely finished with their thought and pause before you respond. First, you will find you are more relaxed in that conversation. Second, you will actually begin to truly understand their point. Third, they will listen to you when you are speaking. You will definitely find that you are far less stressed in a conversation if you actually listen. There will be time in almost all situations to get your point across.

A good communicator has empathy. It is important to put yourself in the other person's position. Try to understand where they are coming from. If you do, you will be in a much better position to understand their point. If there is a disagreement, you are in a much better position to resolve the conflict. The key again is to bring a positive attitude to the situation. Oftentimes, misunderstandings occur because people just are not listening. If there is a question about what the topic is or what the person said, either ask them to repeat their point or say to them, "Can I just rephrase what you said so that I am sure I understood your point?" or, "Is this what you were trying to say?", and state what you heard. You will be surprised how many times that is not what they meant to say or not what they meant for you to understand. It is very hard to be engaged in a conversation when people are actually discussing two different points and they do not realize it. Clearly, this situation leads to a lot of stress. So often, the key is to restate the other person's position. Likewise, it helps to ask the other person to paraphrase your position. This lessens misunderstandings all around and can take the anger out of confrontational situations.

Communication at work can be sometimes difficult. We may be in a position where the boss has spoken to co-workers in a less than empathetic manner. It is important not to take the comments personally. If we have truly made a mistake, we need to understand that mistake and move on. We need to understand what the person we are working for needs us to do. Make sure to understand what they want and review a plan for accomplishing the goal so they are comfortable with the end result. It comes down to clear communication and addressing expectations. We need to check in with our colleagues, coworkers and our boss while we are doing the task. Take responsibility for a positive flow of information. Again, communicate,

communicate, communicate, listen, listen, listen. We have so much to learn from others, and open lines on both ends makes for a much better work atmosphere.

We should try not to be defensive when someone gives us constructive criticism. We may think we do not deserve it, and that we already know what they are telling us, but the potential is there for us to learn something new. We must bring a positive attitude to every conversation.

This does not mean, however, that you become the office doormat! Remember what former First-Lady Eleanor Roosevelt said: "No one can make you feel inferior without your consent". If someone talks down to you or inappropriately accuses you of something you did not do, it is important to stick up for yourself. That does not mean a shouting match in the hallway. You need to state the facts and clearly set the person straight about your part in the situation. You may also say that you are more than happy to be a part of the solution. You need to decide the appropriate time and place for resolving this issue. Often, negative communications are best done one-on-one. Positive communications, such as praising a colleague, boss, friend or family member might be a good situation to share with others. Remember, you are in control of your stress level. Try to keep a positive attitude, even under difficult circumstances. Remember to breathe in slowly, hold your breath for a

> **The Doctor Says...**
>
> "No one can make you feel inferior without your consent".
> - Eleanor Roosevelt

few seconds, and breathe out slowly. Try the old method of counting to ten before you respond in a difficult situation. If you are still not sure about how to handle the situation, call a trusted friend or family member, review it with them and if possible, sleep on it. Oftentimes, you will wake up the next day and know exactly how to handle that difficult situation that seemed almost impossible the day before.

Super Person

Oftentimes, especially with type "A" personalities, we feel we can do anything. We try to cram ten pounds of flour in a five pound bag. Clearly, this will lead to significant stress that we have brought upon ourselves. If we find we constantly do this, we need to do an inventory and discover why we say yes to every request. We 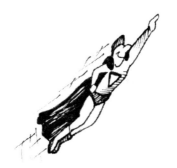 need to realize that it may not be possible to help everyone all the time. It is important that we control our own personal stress, and that we accept responsibilities that are reasonable. It comes back to the time management issue: do we have enough time to do the job well without being completely stressed by the situation? I go back to certain chapters in "Don't Sweat The Small Stuff, It's All Small Stuff" by Richard Carlson. This book has some very straightforward methods of teaching us how to just say no politely. It is important at the beginning of any project to clearly delineate the expectations we have of the people that will be helping us and the expectations that they have with regard to our responsibilities in these tasks. If we do that early in the task, we often will be successful, we will have better time management, less stress, and we will actually enjoy the project.

Anger

When someone says something that enrages us, it is important not to overreact. We may have misunderstood the person or the situation. It is very important to get clarification before we react. The communication skills we learn will help us in these very stressful situations. False accusations and inappropriate expectations must be clarified before we can develop an appropriate response. It is important to keep in mind that we also do not want to deliver a message that will enrage or anger someone else, especially if we do not have the facts.

Anger, over time, will lead to the potential of increased cardiovascular and neurovascular disease, hypertension, poor eating habits and improper sleep patterns, so it is important for us to focus on this.

One of the simplest ways to control anger is to be forgiving. Number one, forgive yourself first. We often get angry with ourselves when we are unable to complete a task. The phrases run through our head; "why did I accept this project", "why did I say yes to this situation". Be a little easier on yourself. No one is 100%, 100% of the time. Also, be forgiving of other people. A little bit of kindness and understanding goes a long way. Empathy makes us happy and helps control our stress. Avoid the dangers of anger, miscommunication, and misunderstanding with our friends, families, and colleagues. Anger, unchecked, can lead to a lot of hurt not only to your own body, your health, your mind, but also to the people around you. Sometimes things are said in anger we wish we had never said. We ask for forgiveness and we need to give it. We also hope that other people will forgive us when we are inappropriate in anger. I have not met anyone in my entire life who has not been inappropriate in anger at some point; we all do it. We need to limit this emotion. We do have the ability to control our emotions, but it is not easy. It requires a lot of effort on our part. There are so many external and internal variables that we deal with constantly, but we strive to have better control of our life and our emotions. Stop blaming yourself for having the inability to control all of your emotional situations. The best we can do is remember that we are responsible for all our behavior, good and bad.

When it comes to a situation of anger and disappointment, it is important to address that issue as soon as is prudently possible with the persons involved. Allowing it to stew for weeks, months, or years will only cause you pain. Find a solution as soon as possible. See Figure 5.

Figure 5

A Solution to Dealing with the Problem of Anger:

1) Write down the issue that made you so angry.
2) Write down the two or three aspects that you feel resulted in this issue developing.
3) Write down several solutions.
4) Write down how you plan to implement the solution you feel is the best, so that this type of situation does not happen again.

Solving a Problem

A simple way to solve a problem can be something as easy as taking out a piece of paper and writing down the problem in one sentence. Then write down in a series of one to two sentences how that problem happened. Then write down two or three potential solutions to that problem. Take the best solution and then write down how you plan to implement that solution and then do it. If it involves just you, you can do it yourself. If it involves other people, then review it with co-workers, family, and friends. Putting it on paper makes you crystallize your thoughts and forces you to think it through. I suggest you use this in every aspect of your life; try it at work. You will discover that you are hardly asking your boss anything; you already figured out the solution. You will become a more efficient worker, realize that you can do these things yourself, increase your confidence, and lower your stress. Another win-win! Writing things down makes you crystallize and focus in ways that just do not happen if you walk around thinking. For most people, this is a very simple and effective solution to many of the problems that are faced in life.

Some problem solving requires research. The internet is one of the best friends you have for getting information. Remember the wisdom of our elders; they have probably faced the same problem that you are now experiencing. Pick up the phone and call your grandparents or parents. Often, you will be pleasantly surprised if you have not used this resource in your life. You will make their day because you have made them useful by letting them know how much you appreciate their wisdom.

Another thing to keep in mind is how big the problem is that one is faced with. Put it in perspective; if this problem is not going to matter a year from now, do not spend a lot of time on it. When you face a really significant problem, if you are religious and believe in God, ask for help, say a prayer, meditate, or take a walk, but come back and commit your thoughts to paper. Sometimes the answer will jump off the page!

Sleep

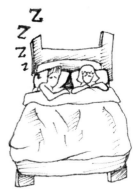

Stress can control sleep. If we are very stressed out by a situation, we often find that we cannot go to sleep. Oftentimes, we will make incorrect choices such as having caffeine or eating a large amount of food late in the day. Then we are too uncomfortable to sleep.

Sleep behavior is very important. Some of the basics seem obvious: avoid caffeinated beverages such as coffee, tea, and some carbonated soft drinks after 1 to 2pm. Avoid foods that contain caffeine (reading labels is helpful here). Certain medicines taken at night may interfere with proper sleep patterns. Alcohol will disrupt sleep as well.

Avoid those really heavy meals at least four hours before bedtime; lighter snacks are much more appropriate. You should try to avoid all significant intake of food 3-4 hours before bedtime.

Remember, the environment of your bedroom needs to be reserved for sleep or loving interactions with your partner; it is not your office or the family entertainment center. Make it your refuge, a place to de-stress.

Make sure the environment is appropriate, the bed is comfortable, the area is appropriately dimmed, and it is quiet. Avoid watching the news, disturbing movies, or playing video games a few hours before bedtime. Also try to avoid exercise 3-4 hours before going to bed.

Should you have continued difficulty with sleep, you actually may have an underlying medical problem such as insomnia or sleep apnea. You may also have a pulmonary, cardiovascular, or neurological problem such as restless leg syndrome. It is important that you seek help from your physician or allied healthcare professional to address this issue further when the simple techniques prove ineffective.

There are many other underlying conditions that disturb sleep. Sometimes excessive worrying, sadness, or anxiety are the result of depression or generalized anxiety disorder, both medical conditions that can be very successfully treated. Depression and anxiety not only can significantly interfere with our sleep pattern, but also significantly interfere with our ability to control stress. It is important when we are not able to manage stress on our own to seek professional help from our physician or allied healthcare professional.

Summary

Stress is change, positive or negative. Ultimately, we choose how to react to stress in our life. Choose a positive attitude; enlist help from your family, friends, and colleagues. Share the good times, share the bad, and when necessary, seek assistance from your physician or allied healthcare professionals and you will be able to manage your stress.

References and Recommended Readings

Davis M, Eshelman E, McKay M. The Relaxation & Stress
    Reduction Workbook. Oakland, CA: New Harbinger
    Publication; 2000. pp 1-286.

Elkin A. Stress Management for Dummies. New York, NY: Wiley
    Publishing: 1999. pp 9-278.

Ferriss T. The 4-Hour Workweek. New York: Crown
    Publishings; 2007. pp 92-98.

Winner J. Stress Management Made Simple. Santa Barbara, CA: Blue
    Fountain Press; 2003. pp 1-151.

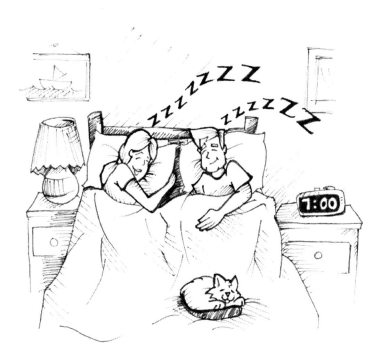

Step 4: Good Sleep Habits

Sleep is not an option; it is a necessity. Most people need 7-8 hours of sleep every night. If you are getting a proper night's rest, you should awaken refreshed and remain alert throughout the day. If this is not the case, there may be something wrong. (Breus, 2006)

Sleep disorders, the most common being sleep apnea, are associated with hypertension, heart disease, stroke, and an increase in automobile, workplace, and household accidents. They can also cause memory problems, anxiety, depression, and increased headaches, especially chronic daily morning headaches. In fact, as many as 50% of individuals suffering from these headaches may actually have an underlying sleep disorder. For years, we have been educating our medical community to look for lesions or brain tumors when diagnosing the causes of morning headaches. More often than not, there is an underlying correctable problem, and a sleep disorder should be seriously considered. If you are waking up tired and feel sluggish throughout the day, or are having morning headaches, it is important to visit your physician or allied healthcare professional.

A lack of sleep for even one night can be associated with difficulty with concentrating, memory, and clear thinking. Should this continue over several nights or more, the situation could be far more serious. Chronic sleeplessness can potentially impair your immune system and increase weight gain, leading to obesity, and a higher incidence of type II diabetes. Many of us simply do not get enough sleep; this is becoming a hidden epidemic in our society. It is time now to pay attention to this disorder.

> **The Doctor Says...**
> Many of us simply do not get enough sleep; this is becoming a hidden epidemic in our society.

Many factors alter the quality of our sleep. One of the most common factors is our use of caffeine. It is fine to have one or two cups of coffee or caffeinated beverages in a day. Most people enjoy it, and it can actually help get us started in the morning! Caffeine is also actually a very good antioxidant; so is green tea, which has less caffeine. For example, a 6-8 ounce cup of coffee will have about 100-110 mg of caffeine. A caffeinated soda or green tea contains about 40-

45 mg of caffeine. It is important to consume your caffeine early in the day, and preferably before 1 to 2 pm.

If you do consume large quantities of caffeine (i.e. six or more cups of coffee or other caffeinated beverages), it is not a good idea to stop abruptly. You want to gradually wean off this high amount of caffeine by dropping one cup (unit) every 7 days. For example, if you are consuming eight cups of coffee a day, decrease to seven cups of coffee for 7 days, then six cups for 7 days, then 5 cups for 7 days, etc. until you are comfortable with drinking only one or two cups daily. Why

> **The Doctor Says...**
> Abrupt withdrawal of caffeine can evoke a withdrawal response.

do I say this? Abrupt withdrawal of caffeine can evoke a withdrawal response. It is quite real, and can last for a week or two. Symptoms include headaches, difficulty concentrating, irritability, mood swings, fatigue, nausea, and even general flu-like symptoms without a fever. It is far better to gradually taper your use of caffeine if you are over utilizing this substance. The most important issue I am raising is why. Why are you using so much caffeine? If you are using it to try to stay awake and alert throughout the day, you need to think about your sleep habits and make changes that will ensure a healthy night's rest. (Breus, 2006)

What other techniques can we use to help alter and improve our sleep patterns? One simple approach is to reduce ambient light. Many of us allow the sun to shine

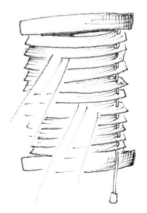

directly into our bedrooms in the morning. That is fine if you actually do get 7-8 hours of sleep before the sun rises. Many of us rise later than the sun. For this reason, it is very important to use appropriate curtains and window treatments to remove ambient bright light. When you are ready to let the morning sun shine in, you open the curtains. If you cannot remove all ambient light, at least place the bed in a position where light is less likely to shine directly on you.

It is also important that your bedroom be set up as a comfortable, quiet room. This may be a challenge if you live in a busy urban environment, but there are some simple solutions like using ear plugs, hanging heavy curtains, and carpeting the room. There are many different ways to make your bedroom soundproof and yet still very pleasing to the eye. **Remember, your bedroom is not the office, the playroom, the family room, and certainly not the dining room!** It is designed and should be utilized solely for the purpose of sleep and sex.

Remove all televisions, and try not to read in bed. Try to remove bright artificial lights from the bedroom. Today, some clocks that are used in the bedroom are quite bright. Try to get a clock that has a very dim component and remove the numbers from your line of vision. Turn the clock in such a way that if you were to look from your bed you cannot see the numbers. It is best to set the alarm and do not worry about it until the alarm goes off; leave it out of your control. If you wake up in the middle of the night, do not worry about the time: go back to sleep; the alarm will go off. If you have a concern and you are in an area where there are power issues, then use a battery backup alarm or a windup alarm.

It is also probably best to avoid allowing your kids and pets to sleep in the bed with you.

It is most important to set aside appropriate time for sleep. Most individuals in the United States just do not get the sleep they need. Consider this as a medical priority for longevity, brain health, and physical health. You will live longer, feel happier and be far more alert if you get a good night's sleep every night. Try to go to bed roughly about the same time every night and get up the same time every morning. For those of us who suffer from migraines, it is absolutely imperative that we keep a very regular sleep schedule. In fact, waking up at the same time can prove quite beneficial in preventing migraine headaches.

> **The Doctor Says...**
> For those of us who suffer from migraines, it is absolutely imperative that we keep a very regular sleep schedule.

There are times when scheduling proper sleep is out of our control, such as traveling for business or pleasure. Do the best you can to get seven or eight hours of sleep. When you change time zones, especially during the first few days, stay outside, get near a window, and try to get as much sunlight as you can. This helps your brain reset your internal clock and get you back to a normal sleep pattern.

Plan ahead when you are traveling. It may be a good idea to bring ear plugs. If you happen to end up being put in the room next to the elevators, or the ice machine, the ear plugs may help soften some of the noise. Should the room not have heavy curtains, or curtains that do not close completely, or you are given a room that faces the sunrise, you may be very unpleasantly awakened early in the morning,

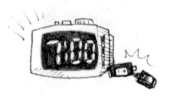 before your scheduled time. To avoid this, bring some clips that will close the gaps in the curtains. They are very inexpensive and lightweight for travel.

Also, consider bringing an eye protector to keep ambient light from waking you early. A battery powered travel alarm clock will alleviate any worries about waking on time for your appointments: you will not need to worry about a wake-up call.

When you find a comfortable hotel or bed and breakfast, try to stay at that same place when you return to that area. Keeping the same environment when traveling can be very comforting, increasing your chance for a good night's sleep. Again, it is imperative that you get some time outside both the day you arrive and the next day to help reset your internal clock. This exposure to light also assists your body to regulate the release of a hormone called melatonin, which is important for proper sleep.

Watch your diet when you are traveling by avoiding heavy meals late at night. Try to keep your diet relatively light. Stay with fruits in the morning and light vegetables without butters or oils. Avoid the heavy greasy, fatty foods completely, if you can, for that evening meal and even for late lunches. Light eating is especially important during the first two days, especially if you are dealing with a significant time change.

If you are having significant difficulty falling asleep when you travel, you may wish to discuss this issue with your doctor or allied healthcare professional. They may recommend using the supplement melatonin or prescription sleep aids. Please do not use medication prescribed for someone else! Discuss this at length with your physician. It is important to use both melatonin and medications appropriately. These are very effective in most individuals, but if used improperly, they could be dangerous. Even something as simple as melatonin, if taken in too large a quantity for too long a period of time, has potentially serious medical side effects, including cardiac arrhythmias at very high doses.

Exercise, as always, is very beneficial. It is best to exercise early in the day and get some exposure to bright sunlight in order to help reset your internal clock, especially when you first arrive. Exercising an hour or two before bed time will increase your metabolic rate and will not help you get to sleep. At night, try to relax at least an hour or so before you are about to go to bed. Some light stretching may be fine. A nice hot bath is always a good idea. Staying up to watch the late night news is not a good way to wind down! Devise a relaxing routine that works for you.

If you find one night that you cannot fall asleep after 15 minutes, do not stay in bed; get up and read or do some relaxing activity until you feel drowsy and then go back to bed.

If at all possible, try not to take the redeye flight. It is better to try to get a good night's sleep and travel the next morning. There are times in our lives when we have no choice, but if it is not a necessity, opt for a different flight. It is not worth saving that time, because the sleep you lose means that you are not going to be as sharp. You are really not saving anything in the long run, and you are possibly hurting yourself. I know from personal experience, redeye flights are really not worth the time you think you save.

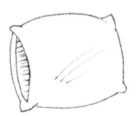 To review, travel with the proper eye covering and ear plugs, think about taking along some soothing music, and bring your own pillow if you find it helps. Planning for your sleep while traveling is important, and will make your trips pleasant and successful. (Breus, 2006)

There are other sleep situations that might leave you somewhat out of control. If your bed partner has restless leg syndrome, they may need medical attention. If he or she snores loudly, medical help is very important. Snoring can potentially be a serious undiagnosed sleep disorder that needs treatment. Anxiety and depression also can influence your sleep patterns rather significantly. Oftentimes, people say they just cannot get to sleep, or conversely that they have no trouble falling asleep, but wake up after a few hours and cannot fall back to sleep. If this is the case, again, please seek help from your physician or allied healthcare professional so that these symptoms can be properly diagnosed and treated.

Other unusual sleep patterns that can occur either in you or in your bed partner are somnambulism (sleep walking), sleep talking, and teeth grinding. Teeth grinding is another sleep problem, and is actually associated with certain types of headache. Many of these problems are correctable, so it is important to get an appropriate evaluation from a health professional. (Victor, 2001)

Again, something as simple as 7-8 hours of sleep every night has the potential to significantly improve the quality of your life, leaving you with the energy and vitality you need throughout the day. It is critically important in maintaining a healthy brain.

For those of you who do have problems with sleep, there are many good books on the market. You need to educate yourself about sleep disorders and proper sleep. I suggest you read "Good Night" by Dr. Michael Breus. It is filled with wonderful insights and suggestions on how to improve the quality of your sleep. This is a great book to begin your education about good sleep habits. Time spent educating yourself about good sleep patterns will be paid back in many years of high quality healthy brain function as well as improved physical stamina, improved quality of life and longevity. Clearly, it is worth the effort.

Key Sleep Issues for a Better Life

It is interesting that as we age, we require different levels of sleep. Infants and young children require more sleep than prior to adolescence. Sleep needs increase again during adolescence. Adults need roughly 7-8 hours a night. I have been discussing the effects of too little sleep: actually it is just as risky to get too much sleep! Long sleepers actually run the risk of increased stroke as well as cardiovascular diseases, depression, and increased risk of diabetes. (Breus, 2006) Again, if you find that you are consistently sleeping 10 or 11 hours nightly, please see a sleep specialist to see if this is normal for you, there could be some underlying problem that could predispose you to more serious medical problems later in your life.

> **The Doctor Says...**
> Adults need roughly 7-8 hours of sleep a night.

If you find yourself sleepy throughout the day, particularly in the late afternoon, sometimes there is a simple solution. Try to get outside into some bright sunlight for about 15 minutes and/or engage in a little physical activity. You may find you can get a brief sense of rejuvenation, and this is a good substitute for a caffeinated beverage.

The most recognized sleep disorders today are insomnia, sleep apnea, narcolepsy and restless leg syndrome. (Kryger, 2005) As we have discussed, many other issues contribute to improper sleep, such as stress, poor diet, and environmental issues. Even your own genetics may predispose you to a potential sleep disorder or to behaviors that will result in poor sleep habits. There are many different ways to approach these disorders and to improve the quality of your sleep, but in most instances if you truly have a sleep disorder that cannot be corrected by some of the simple suggestions of this or other books, it is highly recommended that you seek medical help to get a proper diagnosis and appropriate therapies.

Often, a person or their partner will notice grinding or clenching of their teeth during their sleep. This is called bruxism, and can lead to increased headaches. It is important to get your healthcare professional involved, specifically your dentist, in an effort to maintain proper dental care. Bruxism can damage teeth and lead to potentially more serious issues down the road. There are several simple treatments such as a bite plate worn during sleep. Again, it is imperative you get medical help to address this issue.

Restless leg syndrome or unusual periodic movements of the leg is disturbing for both the sufferer and his/her partner. It is a treatable medical condition and is important for a medical professional to evaluate this problem.

Loud snoring causes many problems for both the snorer and his/her partner. Clearly, the individual with significant snoring is at much greater risk and needs medical attention. Additionally, the individual who is constantly being awakened is not getting the proper sleep. This partner will be predisposed to developing a medical disorder due to the secondary effects of their partner's sleep disorder. (Dement, 1999)

A significant portion of pre-menopausal and menopausal women can experience sleep related disorders, generally noting difficulty with falling asleep and staying asleep. This, of course, results in tiredness and sleepiness throughout the day, and thus decreased alertness and function. Present data suggests that low estrogen/progesterone levels result in increased awakenings in the evening and interference with non-REM sleep. The shifting of hormones in premenopausal and menopausal women can be disruptive to regular sleep patterns. Your physician or healthcare professional will have some suggestions about evaluating and alleviating these symptoms.

Although I am not a proponent of naps as a method of correcting sleep difficulties, they may prove helpful for women who experience lethargy and sleepiness associated with menopausal and premenopausal hormonal fluctuations. There are various supplements that may help such as calcium, magnesium, and B-complex vitamins. Symptoms can also be improved by adjusting exercise, increasing fiber intake in your diet, adding some herbs and spices to your diet, and increasing your antioxidant nutritional intake. (Breus, 2006)

Sleep and Weight Loss

It has become scientifically evident that there is a connection between sleep and the ability to maintain or lose weight. Your body regulates certain chemicals that control hunger and appetite and they are influenced by a lack of sleep. While we are asleep, the body makes the vital chemicals that we need to function properly throughout our day. They help us to control our ability to focus, be alert, deal with stress, improve our creativity, and handle pain. There is also some evidence that these chemicals help maintain good skin texture and allow us to remain more physically youthful. We really do need our "beauty sleep"! However, the aspect of weight management is even more intriguing.

The absolute physics of weight loss and weight maintenance are simple. If you consume more calories than you burn, you gain weight; if you consume less calories than you utilize in a given day, you will eventually lose weight. So how does sleep play in this equation? Here is one very simple observation: while you are sleeping, you cannot eat. Of course, this is only one small piece of a complicated situation. Our hormones play a significant role in our appetite and whether we gain or lose weight. There is a constant delicate balance going on between various hormones in our body. The hormone ghrelin and the hormone leptin are constantly in a ying-yang balance between our feelings of hunger and appetite control. The hormone ghrelin is the hormone that is secreted when our stomach is empty, causing us to experience hunger. If the stomach is full, the hormone leptin is secreted, thus giving the message that we are full and can stop eating. One of the key problems with this system is that it is very slow to react and tell our brain when our stomach is full; there is a lag time. In our fast-paced society, this can result in significant overeating. Added to this societal issue is that if we do not get enough sleep, then this delicate balance between ghrelin and leptin is disrupted. The present information available notes that with decreased sleep, we produce less leptin (which makes us feel full) and thus, increase our production of ghrelin (which makes us feel hungry). This is exactly what we do not want when trying to control or lose weight. If your brain does not get enough leptin, the hormone that makes you feel full, you will continue to feel hungry and you will want to eat. (Breus, 2006) Thus it would seem that lack of sleep directly increases our hunger and cravings for foods that are less than optimum to maintain a healthy brain.

> **The Doctor Says...**
>
> Lack of sleep directly increases our hunger and cravings for foods that are less than optimum to maintain a healthy brain.

You truly need to get a handle on this situation. If this cycle is not interrupted, you ultimately increase your weight. This can result in the development of diabetes type II and significant problems with the regulation of your carbohydrate metabolism, leading to many of the health disorders we have already discussed. It is absolutely vital that you get the proper amount of sleep you need on a daily basis. Even subtle disruptions of sleep over just a few weeks, can result in abnormalities of the metabolism of carbohydrates and abnormal regulation of blood sugar and production of insulin, ultimately predisposing you to the future development of diabetes type II.

We humans have an extremely complex neuroendocrine system containing multiple checks and balances in an effort to maintain proper metabolism. One of these checks is the growth hormone which also influences the delicate balance between carbohydrates, fats, and proteins and how they are metabolized in our body. How sleep influences the regulation of the growth hormone must also be addressed.

The final two hormones we will discuss are cortisol and serotonin. They are delicately balanced and are closely linked to sleep and weight maintenance. Cortisol has been discussed in relation to stress management. When you are under significant or chronic stress, cortisol is released, resulting in increased appetite and hunger, thus driving individuals to eat excessively. From this feeling comes the popularity of "comfort foods" which often contain high carbohydrate and fructose corn syrup levels. Cortisol levels are lowest during our sleep state and highest when we awaken in the morning. (Breus, 2006)

Another consequence of sleeplessness is a lack of production and release of serotonin. This is a very important compound. There are more serotonin receptors than any other receptor. They are found in a high degree in the brain and in smaller quantities throughout the entire body, especially in the intestinal tract. Serotonin is associated with pain control, mood, and depression. Inadequate amounts of this compound may lead people again to seek "comfort foods" in an effort to control their mood or their depressive feelings, thus resulting again in eating the wrong foods to excess. The study of neuroendocrinology, the interplay of these various hormones, is vital and I suggest you read as much as you can on this topic. Discuss this with your physician and allied healthcare professional. They should be able to provide you with many sources of information related to these topics. The more you understand about how these hormones interact and how sleep is vital in the control of these hormones, the easier it will be for you to maintain your ideal body weight (a BMI between 18 and 24.9). It will be easier for you to handle a diet when you understand why you have these cravings and why you are always hungry, and it will help you make better choices when it comes to appropriate brain nutrition and brain supplementation.

What about Naps?

Are naps beneficial? Like most things in medicine, the answer depends on the individual. Although we focused on the importance of 7-8 hours of sleep a night, some people function well with less sleep, and some feel better by napping. It is felt by most clinicians that routine daily napping is not a good idea; however, some of us actually do well with an afternoon nap. Let us discuss a few nap issues.

Different nap time periods actually have potentially different influences on your brain.

Some clinicians believe that naps are actually beneficial and might possibly lower the risk of cardiovascular or neurovascular disease. They may also help in stabilizing our mood, our attitude, and increase productivity, but more research needs to be done before an indisputable conclusion can be made.

If you find yourself excessively tired, have trouble staying alert, or having some difficulty with memory in the afternoon, a nap may prove beneficial to you. A brief nap can result in increased alertness, improved memory retention, and a sense of well being. It may even result in sharpening your motor skills. If you are driving a car and feel less alert, clearly it is imperative that you pull over and take a brief rest, go for a walk, or even take a brief nap before you proceed.

If you consider taking a nap, a "power nap" is roughly about a 20 minute time period. Naps can be as short as five minutes or as long as 2-3 hours. It is suggested not to exceed three hours because this might disrupt your evening sleep.

> **The Doctor Says...**
>
> If you consider taking a nap, a "power nap" is roughly about a 20 minute time period.

The actual optimum time for a nap is really an individual matter. A nap lasting somewhere between 30 minutes to one hour is reasonable and is best usually about eight hours after you awaken. If you wake up and you are groggy and non-refreshed then this is not the optimum time, and you need to adjust the time until you actually do wake refreshed, more alert, and ready for the activities of the rest of the day.

Should you wake up from a nap feeling groggy and listless, you may be able to bring yourself back to alertness rather quickly by washing your face in cold water, going for a brisk walk for about 10-15 minutes, or listening to some invigorating and stimulating music. These activities will help resynchronize your brain function and bring you back to an alert functioning state. (Breus, 2006)

Your Sleep Cycle

A few words on the sleep cycle may help you understand the above recommendations.

Sleep happens in various stages. Machines that monitor sleep show that our brain is extremely active during these stages. Stage one is the initial stage where we are a little drowsy and we drift off into sleep. Initially the brain goes from an alpha, or the awake state, to a mixed theta or drowsy state, which is stage two or light sleep. This is the sequence of the power nap. It is easy to awaken from a stage two sleep and feel refreshed. If we stay asleep, we will transition to a deeper sleep with delta wave activity. Stages three and four show slow wave activity on an EEG(which measures and records the electrical activity of the brain, much like an electrocardiogram measures and records the electrical activity of the heart), making it more difficult to wake up, leaving you groggy and listless. Stage five is referred to as REM sleep, the dream state. Often your eyes will twitch, but your body is somewhat paralyzed; you do not move during this stage of sleep, but your brain is extremely active during this time. This is a very important stage of restorative sleep. During stages three, four, and five, significant metabolic mechanisms are taking place with the release of hormones, specifically growth hormone, and the production of various proteins, enzymes, and other hormones that are going to be needed for the next day.

It is felt that stage five sleep is extremely important in learning and the ability to retain and process information. The old saying "I will sleep on it" may have scientific validity. It would seem that during this stage of sleep we actually work out some of our lingering problems and come up with solutions. I am sure you have experienced this phenomenon: you went to bed with a problem and woke up the next day with an incredibly brilliant solution. Your brain has worked through the night to come up with solutions to help you during the next day.

> **The Doctor Says...**
> Your brain has worked through the night to come up with solutions to help you during the next day.

These five stages of sleep repeat over and over throughout the evening, but they do vary subtly. In the earlier stages of the evening, they tend to be shorter, around 80 minutes and then they expand and lengthen later in the evening up to about 120 minutes, cycling on average 4-6 times in normal individuals.

Doctors are now paying a lot more attention to this fascinating research about normal sleep patterns as well as sleep related disorders. Over the coming years and decades, we will clearly become far more enlightened about the importance of sleep as it relates to maintaining a healthy brain. (Kryger, 2005)

Summary

There are some straight-forward approaches to maintaining good health with proper sleep. The most important of all is to get 7-8 hours of sleep every night. If you cannot do that, or if you still wake up non-refreshed and are not alert during the day, you need to determine whether you have an underlying sleep disorder or other medical disorder that is preventing a proper night's rest. I cannot emphasize this point enough in this chapter. Again, see your physician or allied healthcare professional to get this situation corrected.

Simply stated, the proper amount of sleep leads to an appropriate balance between hunger and satiation, appropriate metabolism, and the appropriate maintenance of our weight. Lack of sleep for more than just a few days will result in disruption of the systems controlling our hunger along with our metabolism, leading to potential increased weight gain.

I would additionally like to say just a few words about aging and our skin. Some really simple ways to have younger skin are to avoid excessive sun exposure, use appropriate sunscreens to block damaging UVA and UVB rays, avoid smoking, control your weight, keep your BMI between 18 and 24, and get a good night's sleep. Ultimately it will lead to a healthier brain and a healthier body, resulting in a more youthful appearance: when you feel good, you look good!

References and Recommended Reading

Breus M. Good Night. New York, NY: Dutton; 2006. pp1-311.

Dement W. The Promise of Sleep. New York, NY: Dell
Publishing; 1999. pp1- 470.

Kryger M, Roth T, Dement W. Principles and Practice of Sleep
Medicine. Philadelphia, PA: 2005. pp 39-888.

Victor M,Ropper AH. Principles of Neurology. New
York, NY: McGraw-Hill; 2001. pp 404-427.

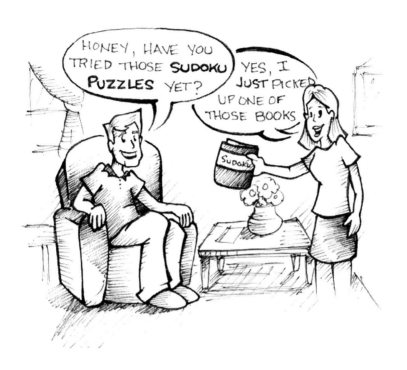

Step 5: Exercise the Brain

There is an old saying, "use it or lose it". It is actually true when it comes to the brain. If we do not exercise our brain, it will atrophy. Our brain is not a muscle, but there are some similarities. If you do not use a muscle, it will atrophy and you will physically see it shrink. If you do not use your brain, you will not physically see the brain shrink, [without the aid of neuroimaging equipment (CT scan or MRI)], but you will intellectually suffer and experience a cognitive decline. *We cannot stick our brain on a treadmill or put it on a bicycle, but we can exercise our brain.* We can improve the function of the most important organ in our body.

Your brain, as an adult, is made up of more than 100 BILLON nerve cells with more than 100 TRILLON (100,000,000,000,000) connections (synapses). The nerve impulses in your brain can travel at speeds greater than 250 miles per hour, amazing. The more synaptic connections your brain forms, the healthier and more powerful you become. The key is to exercise your brain in order to increase the synaptic connections; thus, keeping your brain younger.

> **The Doctor Says...**
> As we age into late adulthood we could be losing up to 100,000 brain cells a day due to cell death.

As we age into late adulthood, we could be losing up to 100,000 brain cells a day due to cell death (free radical damage, wear and tear). This results in the atrophy of your brain. There is a thinning of the outer layer of the brain (cortex) and an enlargement of the fluid filled spaces (ventricles). This tissue loss is more noticeable in the frontal and temporal lobes (front and sides) of the brain. There is also potential deterioration in the blood supply of the brain due to deposits of plaque that build up inside the blood vessels and restrict blood flow. This situation results in sapping us of the vital nutrients (potential energy) we need to help us think and maintain a healthy brain.

The brain communicates by generating electricity, an energy consuming process; this is why the brain requires so much energy each day. This is also why it is so important to give the brain the highest quality food and supplements daily to help maintain a healthy brain.

Memory

Your brain has an extraordinary capacity to store information at all ages. Memory is a store of information that requires a strengthening of connection between neurons. The process involves increasing the number of synaptic connections between the appropriate interconnected neurons. Information is initially stored as short-term memory (about 30 seconds). Significant information is then transferred to long-term memory (stored from hours to years); this process is called consolidation. Different strategies to maximize your memory include: repeating information over and over (repetition is the mother of learning), drawing a mental map (picture), and multimodal, for example, writing a list and then reading it out loud. (Fellows, 2002)

When we perceive that we are beginning to lose our memory, we often ask ourselves if this is normal for age or a symptom of depression, a small stroke, or early Alzheimer's dementia. Most early memory lapses are not due to the above disorders, especially in the younger adult individuals. An occasional lapse in memory, forgetting to pick up something at the store or misplacing an item at home, is felt to be a normal part of life at any age. Some people may suffer from memory problems due to deficiencies in their diets, especially a deficiency in the B vitamins.

Proper levels of neurotransmitters (brain chemicals) are vital for the brain to function normally. If the brain does not have the proper levels of neurotransmitters it will begin to malfunction. It is important that the body be provided the proper nutrients to manufacture adequate amounts of neurotransmitters. (Balch, 2006)

> ## The Doctor Says...
> There are numerous factors that can adversely affect memory loss.

There are numerous factors that can adversely affect memory loss that include: free radical damage, stress, thyroid disorders, and hypoglycemia, to name a few. Unfortunately, age is the key risk factor for the development of dementia. The number of patients that will receive the diagnosis of Alzheimer's dementia doubles every five years in the elderly population.

Although Alzheimer's dementia is the most common form of dementia, other differentials need to be considered. These include multi-infarct dementia (multiple strokes), Frontotemporal dementia, Pick's disease, and Alcoholic and Creutzfeldt-Jakob disease (CJD). The brain of an Alzheimer's patient is characterized by atrophy with destructive plaques and tangles in the neuronal structure, resulting in a marked reduction in the neurotransmitter levels especially acetylcholine. Individuals who stay mentally active tend to be more resistant to develop the clinical signs of dementia. It would seem these individuals continue to make new neuronal synaptic connections while others are being lost; thus, mental stimulation may help to delay cognitive decline. (Fellows, 2002)

In general, as we age, people tend to find it more difficult to learn new information and recall memories. By exercising the brain by focusing on different aspects of brain function, we can maintain or improvement our brain fitness. (Fellows, 2002)

Mental challenges in multiple domains are necessary to maintain a healthy brain. There are many ways to exercise your brain and have fun at the same time. These mental challenges can consist of some simple things like 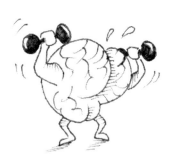 crossword puzzles, word juggles, math games, Sudoku, and board games. (Vorderman, 2005) (Gordon, 2006) (Shortz, 2006) If you like these, you should do them as frequently as you like, preferably one or two of these every day. Challenge your brain constantly. It will lead you to a healthier and more vibrant brain function.

Another option to exercise the brain is to learn a new language. You can learn a new language, travel to the country, and be able to speak the native language and interact with the people, what an incredible use of your brain.

Additionally, something as simple as a board game with your family can exercise your brain and allow you to have a great time. Easy ideas like this should be incorporated into your regular routine.

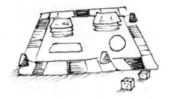

Other options include playing card games, such as Bridge or poker. If you do not know how to play Bridge, then I recommend you learn.

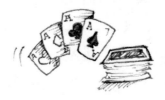

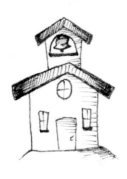

Go to school, take classes, and meet new people. Enroll in a course on a subject matter you always wanted to study; take the time to find a high school or college night course that you find interesting. They are easy to find, they are everywhere, and they are very enjoyable. Again, you meet new people, find new friends, and do something you have always wanted to do.

As we get older, it is important that we increase the amount of mental exercises we do. As people get older, especially people who are approaching retirement, the idea is not to use your brain less. It is important to use your brain for things that you have wanted to use it for that you may not have had the chance to, such as the examples above. Learn a new language, take some new courses, or learn to play a game you really are not familiar with.

It is important to increase your mental processing as you age, in an effort to retard the natural aging process, which I must add is actually in dispute when it comes to the brain. There is a decline in cognitive function that can begin as early as 30 years of age, but is this decline normal for humans or is it the beginnings of underlying neuropathology? Pathology that we now diagnose in 60, 70, and 80 year olds as memory disorders, Alzheimer's, and dementia. Could the decline in the 30's be an early sign of

> **The Doctor Says...**
> By taking appropriate steps, we can slow down the aging process and possibly reverse it.

impending dementia that we may be able to pick up and treat earlier, or is it normal cognitive decline because we are not exercising our brain properly when we are young? Currently, we are aging much faster than we should be, and by taking appropriate steps, we can slow down the aging process and possibly reverse it. Further research is needed to address these issues.

The structural and functional decline that accompanies aging from age thirty to beyond eighty includes the decline of brainwaves and volume anywhere from 10-20%, as well as a decline in a number of nerve fibers that can be as great as 35%. Again, we know there is a volume loss that occurs and that seems to be accepted by all scientists as a normal aging process. What is not accepted by all scientists is that the decline in nerve fibers is normal as we age. Many of us feel that with the data that is available at this point, it is not normal to lose large quantities of nerve cells as we age. The loss of these significant numbers of nerve cells is actually an indication of an underlying neurological disorder for which we must diagnosis and treat early. Either way, we are seeing a loss of nerve cells in a large part of our population as they pass the age of thirty.

We must do everything possible to slow this process down. This process can be slowed down by the use of proper medical care, proper evaluations, and in the future, hopefully, we will be able to use genetics to help us figure out who is at risk and take effective preventive steps. Today, it is important that you exercise your brain; begin immediately if you have not already done so in a significant way.

As we age, our ability to remember, memorize, acquire new knowledge and recall names does seem to diminish, but we can help to retard this decline.

We know that aging begins when free radical damage occurs at the cellular level and damages DNA; thus, the use of antioxidants can help to prevent this destruction. Proper brain nutrition and proper brain supplementation are vital components in the process to help maintain optimum brain function.

Careful study has shown us that surviving neurons, as we age, can respond to the cell loss and develop new synaptic connections in an effort to preserve functions. Synaptic connections are a method by which nerve cells communicate with each other, and it is important that we maintain proper synaptic function so that we can remember, recall, and learn. This means that your brain will be able to regenerate if given the proper tools. The brain is able to do this with proper exercise. There is a decline in the concentration of neurotransmitters as we

The Doctor Says...

Your brain will be able to regenerate if given the proper tools.

age. This decline in neurotransmitters includes acetylcholine (very important in memory), norepinephrine, dopamine, serotonin, and gamma aminobutyric acid (GABA). These are all vital to maintaining proper brain function.

The nerve cells you are born with must last your entire life since, to the best of our knowledge, our nerve cells do not divide. If a nerve cell dies, it is destroyed forever. If a nerve cell dies by aging, trauma, or disease, it is not coming back; it is not replaced. It is important that we protect every single nerve cell in our brain everyday as adults.

Prevention is the key to the preservation of a healthy brain. By the way, alcohol in moderation would seem to be fine for most individuals. However, significant amounts of alcohol consumed daily, over many years, can result in significant shrinkage and loss of brain cells, due to destruction and death of those cells. Moderation is key in many situations in life, especially when it comes to the use of alcohol.

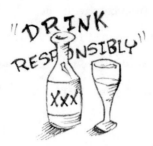

Summary

It takes 25 years in some individuals to fully develop the human brain. It is felt by some neuroscientists that little new or original development is initiated by the brain after age forty. They feel that high intellect, well organized work habits, and sound judgment compensate for the progressive deficiencies of aging. The effects of aging on brain function seem extremely variable among individuals. (Victor, 2001) There is continued maintenance of the brain structure needed every single moment of your life. Utilize all of the seven steps to help you maintain optimum brain function.

References and Recommended Readings

Breus M. Good Night. New York, NY: Dutton; 2006. pp. 1-283.

Balch PA. Prescription for Nutritional Healing. 4th ed. New York, NY: Avery Penguin Group; 2006. pp. 3-807.

Fellows L. the Brain and Central Nervous System. Reader's Digest Association, Inc.: Pleasantville, NY; 2002. Pp 8-155.

Gordon P, Longo F. Mensa Guide to Solving Sudoku. New York, NY: Sterling Publishing Co., Inc.; 2006. pp.5-271.

Pizzorno JE, Murray M. Textbook of Natural Medicine. 3rd ed. St. Louis, Missouri: Churchill Livingstone Elsevier; 2006. pp. 709-2201.

Roizen MF, Oz MC. You on a Diet. New York, NY: Free Press; 2006. pp.3-354.

Shortz W, Maleska ET. The New York Times Supersized Book of Sunday Crosswords. New York, NY: St. Martin's Griffin; 2006. pp 1-500.

Victor M, Ropper AH. Adams and Victor's Principles of Neurology. 7th ed. New York: McGraw-Hill Medical Publishing Division; 2001 pp. 45-1644.

Vorderman C. Master Sudoku. New York, NY: Three Rivers Press; 2005. pp 4-320.

Winner P, Lewis DW, Rothner AD. Headache in Children and Adolescents 2nd ed. Hamilton, Ontario: BC Decker, Inc.; 2008. pp. 1-314.

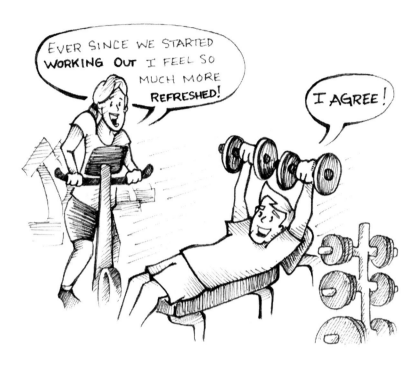

Step 6: Exercise the Body

Physical exercise is imperative to maintaining and improving healthy brain function, focusing, and concentrating. It improves your processing speed and your working memory. It is amazing how a simple exercise program can dramatically improve your health, mood, and life.

The number one reason for physical exercise is to lengthen and strengthen the quality of your brain function and your life.

What do you have to do to achieve this? An effective exercise program includes 30-60 minutes of exercise; for example, one can fast walk at least five or six times a week. (Roizen, 2006) *Your exercise program should include a proper stretching routine both before you start your main exercises and after you complete your main exercises.*

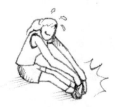

Stretching is an effective way to decrease injury and minimize muscle discomfort. The performance of regular stretching will improve your range of motion, increase muscle strength, help to reduce fatigue, improve posture, promote circulation, improve relaxation and increase energy. If you want to study this subject matter in detail, I recommend you read the book "Fitness & Health", written by Brian Sharkey and Steven Gaskill, and the text "The Anatomy of Stretching", written by Brad Walker. Doctors Roizen and Oz, in their book "You on a Diet", have wonderfully illustrated sections on this issue that I highly recommend you review.

The Doctor Says...
Exercise has been shown to reduce the normal shrinkage of the brain.

Exercise has been shown to reduce the normal shrinkage of the brain, specifically the frontal cortex and the executive functioning area. These two areas control intelligence. Additionally, exercise can also help to prevent stroke, cardiovascular, neurovascular, and peripheral vascular disease issues. (Pizzorno, 2006)

Furthermore, *exercise is associated with reduction of Alzheimer's.* As we diagnose it, people at age seventy who exercise through their adult years can reduce their risk of getting Alzheimer's up to 30 percent. (Balch, 2006)

Continuous activity and proper physical fitness, without question, lowers the risk of cardiovascular, neurovascular, and peripheral vascular disease, specifically stroke, heart attacks, hypertension, peripheral emboli, and loss of limbs resulting in amputation, especially in diabetics type II. (Schlosberg, 2005)

Why is it important to exercise with regards to our brain?

It is important for all aspects of our nervous system to exercise appropriately. We do see that people who exercise consistently seem to have a significantly better ability to control both neck and back pain, and if they do get injured, they are less likely to require a significant recovery period. These people use less medicine and they have a much better quality of life. (Pizzorno, 2006)

We must have a regular routine of exercise. It is important to vary that routine; people get bored if they do the same exercise over and over again. Some exercises may be inside and some may be outside. I urge you to use a gym, go for a walk, bicycle, or swim.

Different times of the year will allow you to do different exercises, so vary your routines.

> **The Doctor Says...**
> It is also important to include weight training as part of your overall fitness plan.

It is also important to include weight training as part of your overall fitness plan. Bone loss can begin as early as your thirties. Lifting weights can hold or reverse this situation, so it is important to exercise your whole body. Physical exercise is almost as important, if not more important, than brain exercising techniques to keep the brain properly functioning. Proper strengthening has to be part of your overall workout.

> **The Doctor Says...**
> Exercise will give you more energy, period.

People sometimes say they cannot exercise, and just do not have enough energy. Well as we have discussed in other chapters, there are many aspects of the seven steps that need to be implemented to help you with improved energy. Exercise will give you more energy, period.

Focused exercise can strengthen the abdomen, the lower back area, and lead to improvement of chronic lower back discomfort. In many patients, losing weight and strengthening the abdomen has resulted in a significant decreased use of medication to control back pain. Again, supplements and good nutrition will help you to obtain pain relief.

Regular exercise can reduce the risk of the development of heart disease, hypertension, diabetes, colon cancer, breast cancer, and even benign prostatic hypertrophy.

Exercise helps you fall asleep faster and stay asleep longer. People who exercise regularly spend more time in slow wave sleep, that is, the restorative state of sleep that you need to wake up rested and alert, staying alert throughout the day. (Schlosberg, 2005)

When is the best time to exercise?

It is important to exercise early in the day. Try to exercise when you first get up; if you cannot, try to exercise before the evening. It is not a good idea to exercise a couple of hours before bedtime, because you will increase your metabolic rate and make it more difficult for you to fall asleep. (Breus, 2006)

The other good reason for exercising early in the day is that you increase your metabolic rate early in the morning, so you are less likely to overeat throughout the day. You are going to be more efficient in the utilization of the food that you do eat and you will be less hungry when you eat. In general, you improve the quality of your life every single day. (Roizen, 2006)

Protect your brain at all times during exercise. It is recommended to wear proper certified bicycle helmets when cycling. It makes no sense to be exercising, get hit by a car and get significant brain damage when you are exercising primarily to improve

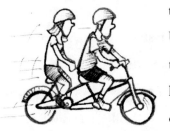

the quality of your brain function. Unfortunately, I have seen this and had to treat many patients who have been hit by cars or fallen off bicycles due to obstacles in the road. They had significant neurological damage from this trauma, some irreversible. These were clearly completely preventable situations, in most instances, had they just worn a certified bicycle helmet. Also, be sure you put the helmet on properly. A lot of individuals do not properly adjust the helmet and as such, in a fall, it does not deliver the full protection that it could have. When engaging in team sports or individual sports where wearing a helmet is appropriate, make sure to use high quality certified head gear to protect your brain. Whether it is football, lacrosse, or even downhill skiing or snowboarding, wear protective head gear. (Winner, 2008)

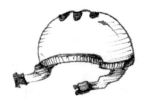

Summary

So what are you waiting for? Join a local gym, find a workout buddy, or go on a walk with your spouse or pet. Get out there and start exercising; it is fun and the benefits are great! Physical exercise is imperative in order to maintain a healthy brain and a healthy body.

References and Recommended Readings

Breus M. Good Night. New York, NY: Dutton; 2006. pp1-283.

Balch PA. Prescription for Nutritional Healing. 4th ed. New York, NY: Avery Penguin Group; 2006. Pp 3-807.

Pizzorno JE, Murray M. Textbook of Natural Medicine. 3rd ed. St. Louis, Missouri: Churchill Livingstone Elsevier; 2006. pp 709-2201.

Roizen MF, Oz MC. You on a Diet. New York, NY: Free Press; 2006 pp 3-354.

Schlosberg S, Neporent L. Fitness for Dummies. Hoboken, NJ: Wiley Publishing, Inc.; 2005. pp1-392.

Sharkey BJ, Gaskill SE. Fitness & Health. 6th ed. Champaign, IL: Human Kinetics; 2007. pp1-400.

Victor M, Ropper AH. Adams and Victor's Principles of Neurology.

7th ed. New York: McGraw-Hill Medical Publishing Division; 2001. pp 45-1644.

Walker B. The Anatomy of Stretching. Chichester, England: Lotus Publishing; 2007. pp 11-165.

Winner P, Lewis DW, Rothner AD. Headache in Children and Adolescents 2nd ed. Hamilton, Ontario: BC Decker, Inc.; 2008 pp1-314.

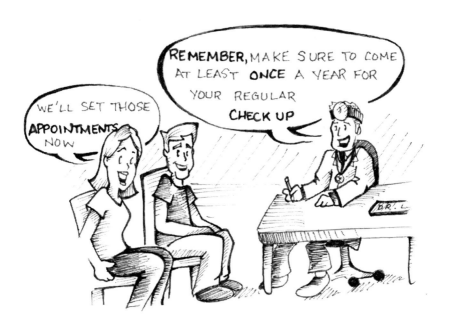

Step 7: Timely Medical Evaluations

It is suggested in today's medical climate that, if at all possible, you **_establish yourself with a primary care physician or primary allied healthcare professional that you can grow old with_**. That person gets to know you, and you get to know that healthcare professional. Establish a personal medical relationship with this individual so that when you do have a medical condition, they can recognize right away that you are not yourself. However, for many people, they tell me, "I cannot do this; my health plan keeps changing, who I can see?" Know you can help this. You decide who you will see. You may have to adjust your financial situation in such a way that you may have to pay from time-to-time to see a specific person, or insist on staying with a healthcare plan that allows you to see that

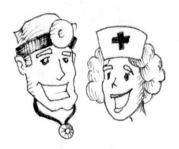

person. Your health insurance plan is your personal life insurance while you are alive! It is absolutely imperative that you have healthcare personnel who know you; they know when you are well and can easily tell when you are ill,

even before you can. You want to work with someone to prevent neurological and cardiovascular disorders from occurring in the first place. If they do occur, you want them to be recognized early and slow down there progression. ***This could actually mean your life, or the life of a loved one, could be saved.***

If you follow these simple suggestions, you and your family have the potential to live a long and happy life. Why have regular physical exams and interact with your healthcare professional? Because it is not unreasonable for you to live a long, healthy, productive, and active life past age 100. Some basic premises are that individuals who are between 30 and 40 get a physical exam at least once every two years; yearly is even better. If you are over 40, regular exams on a yearly basis are strongly recommended. Now, if you say your medical insurance does not allow exams that frequently, then it is necessary to allocate an appropriate amount of your financial resources to keep your brain and body healthy. At certain intervals, other interventional studies will be necessary as part of a comprehensive preventive healthcare plan; colonoscopy is a good example of this. A colonoscopy may be suggested earlier than general recommendations if you have a family history of colon cancer. These are just some of the many reasons why you must establish a good relationship with your primary healthcare professional.

It is also important that you become involved in your own healthcare; you need to understand what is normal and what should be done at various medical visits. One of these issues today is cholesterol; you should know the difference between HDL and LDL. You should know the importance of triglycerides. You should know what metabolic syndrome is and how it is different than diabetes type II. (See Glossary)

If this is all new to you, then you need to start reading. You need to start asking your healthcare professional to give you materials to read. You need to start utilizing appropriate websites that  are peer reviewed by physicians or allied healthcare professionals. Peer reviewed websites can be used to educate patients about good medical health, potential illnesses, and where to get more information.

Education, education, education, I cannot stress this enough. It is good to exercise your brain by reading. You need to learn this to protect yourself and your loved ones by knowing to seek medical care. Through knowledge, you get the earliest and most accurate diagnosis, and are given the appropriate treatment options.

It is important today to utilize the Seven Steps, a concept of utilizing appropriate medical intervention, both prevention and treatment, when nervous system and body medical illnesses occur. An effective integrated approach for the treatment of neurological disorders combines traditional pharmacology with supplements and when needed, physical therapy and/or behavioral therapy.

Utilize the 7 steps of nutrition, supplementation, proper sleep, stress management, and proper exercises of the brain and body. Implement these 7 steps in your life to improve and maintain a healthy brain and body.

If there is any concern with regard to an abnormality in your bodily functions or brain function, especially relating to the nervous system, the results may be very unforgiving. If you lose a nerve cell, it is lost forever, so we must preserve every nerve cell we possibly can as an adult. It is imperative that you seek help early; do not sit on a neurological disorder. Even if it turns out

> **The Doctor Says...**
> It is imperative that you seek help early; do not sit on a neurological disorder.

to be nothing, it is still important to get help, ask questions, and see your doctor. If your doctor cannot help you, get a second opinion; see a neurologist or neurosurgeon for a neurological disorder.

Every step of the seven steps is important. For some of us, one step will be more important than another in any given part in our life. All the seven steps are necessary, and although one may have more weight than another at any given time, they all are equally weighted over our lifetime. Utilize the concepts in the Seven Steps to a Healthy Brain, not as a solution and end-all, but as a beginning to learn about these issues, to educate yourself, and to become more inquisitive. I highly urge you to educate yourself on the concepts in this book and then educate others. Use your healthcare professionals and your physicians to help educate yourself. Remember that neither I, nor any other physician or healthcare professional, has all of the answers. We are constantly learning new material every single day. We are constantly realizing that what we thought was absolutely true today, may not be tomorrow. It is important to question yourself, to question your physician, and to question the data that we have available.

Summary

Remember to work with your physician and/or healthcare professionals; they want to help you. There are a lot of good physicians and healthcare professionals doing incredible research in the field of neuroscience throughout the world, trying to solve the problems that we are addressing in the Seven Steps. Significant headway is being made across the board in the fields of headache, migraine, memory disorder, Alzheimer's, sleep disorders, vascular disease, stroke, cardiovascular disease that may influence brain function, problems with back pain that plague many of us, and general pain syndromes, all of which are under significant study today. Breakthroughs are occurring every single day at different levels.

Physicians are realizing the importance of nutrition, supplementation, and exercise as part of an overall comprehensive medical management system. Sleep is getting more attention. It is so vital that we get a proper, good, restful night sleep, since that alone can help improve medical conditions and prevent disease. (Breus, 2006)

I again suggest that you utilize the information offered to you by your own healthcare professionals. I also suggest that you visit www.DrWinner.org/InsiderResources and sign up for the free newsletter only available for my readers. This exclusive newsletter will give you timely updates about the Seven Steps and inform you as breakthroughs in neuroscience occur.

I leave you with this thought:

People SEE but they do not LOOK,
People HEAR but they do not LISTEN,
People TOUCH but they do not FEEL.

Learn to LOOK, LISTEN, and FEEL everyday
to maintain a Healthy Brain.

Dr. Paul Winner

References and Recommended Readings

Breus M. Good Night. New York, NY: Dutton; 2006.pp 1-283.

Balch PA. Prescription for Nutritional Healing. 4th ed. New York, NY: Avery Penguin Group; 2006. pp 3-807.

Pizzorno JE, Murray M. Textbook of Natural Medicine. 3rd ed. St. Louis, Missouri: Churchill Livingstone Elsevier; 2006. pp 709-2201.

Victor M, Ropper AH. Adams and Victor's Principles of Neurology. 7th ed. New York: McGraw-Hill Medical Publishing Division; 2001 pp 45-1644.

Winner P, Lewis DW, Rothner AD. Headache in Children and Adolescents 2nd ed. Hamilton, Ontario: BC Decker, Inc.; 2008 pp1-314.

Glossary

Adenosine Triphosphate(ATP) - high energy compound formed from oxidation of fat and carbohydrate and used as energy supply for muscle and other body functions.

Allergy - an unusually high sensitivity to normally harmless substances such as pollens, food, or microorganisms. Common symptoms include sneezing, itching, eye irritation and rashes.

Alternative Therapy - the treatment of disease by means other than conventional medical, pharmacological, and surgical techniques.

Amino Acids - chief components of proteins; different arrangements of the 22 amino acids form the various proteins (muscles, enzymes, hormones).

Analgesic - tending to relieve pain, or a substance that relieves pain.

Antibiotic - a substance or drug used to treat infections originally derived from fungi, bacteria, and other organisms.

Antioxidants - substances, such as beta-carotene and vitamins C and E, which block or inhibit oxidation within cells. Antioxidants may reduce the risks of cancer and slow the progression of age-related macular degeneration.

Arteriosclerosis - a circulatory disorder characterized by a thickening and stiffening of the walls of large and medium sized arteries, which impedes circulation.

Ascorbate - a mineral salt of Vitamin C. Taken as nutritional supplements, ascorbates as less acidic (and therefore less irritating) than pure ascorbic acid and also provide for better absorption of both the vitamin C and the mineral.

Ascorbic acid - the organic acid more commonly known as vitamin C.

Atherosclerosis - narrowing of coronary arteries by cholesterol buildup within the walls.

Aura - a subjective sensation that precedes an attack of migraine or epilepsy. With epilepsy, it may precede the actual attack by hours or seconds, and may be of a psychic nature of sensory with olfactory, visual, auditory, or taste hallucinations. In a migraine attack, the aura immediately precedes the attack and primarily consists of visual sensory phenomena.

Bacteria - single celled microorganisms. Some can cause disease, other bacteria are normally present in the body and perform such useful functions as aiding digestion and protecting the body from harmful invading organisms.

Benign - harmless, used to refer to cells, especially cells growing in inappropriate locations, that are not malignant (cancerous).

Beta-carotene - a substance the body uses to make vitamin A.

Biofeedback - a technique for helping an individual to become conscious of usually unconscious body processes, such as heartbeat or body temperature, so that he or she can gain some measure of control over them, and thereby learn to manage the effects of various disorders, including acute back pain, and migraines.

Bioflavonoid - any of a group of biologically active flavonoids. They are essential for the stability and absorption of vitamin C. Although they are not technically vitamins, they are sometimes referred to as Vitamin P.

Biotin - a component of the B-vitamin complex formerly designated vitamin H. This is a water soluble substance important in the metabolism of fats and carbohydrates. Preset in many foods, it is particularly found in the liver, kidney, mild, egg yolks, and yeast.

Blood Count - a basic diagnostic test in which a sample of blood is examined and the number of red blood cells, white blood cells, and platelets determined; or the results of such a test.

Blood Sugar - the glucose, a form of sugar, present in the blood.

Blood-Brain Barrier - a mechanism involving the capillaries and certain other cells of the brain that keeps many substances, especially water-based substances, from passing out of the blood vessels to be absorbed by the brain tissue.

Body Mass Index - A common method using weight and height to estimate overweight, obesity, and risk for chronic diseases such as heart disease, stroke, hypertension, hyperlipidemia, and diabetes. The index is calculated as weight in kilograms divided by height in meters squared (kg/m2).

Calorie Cost - the energy expenditure in calories of an activity. Usually measured in calories per minute.

Calorie - amount of heat required to raise 1 kilogram of water 1 degree Celsius, same as kilocalorie.

Carbohydrate - Simple (e.g. sugar) and complex (e.g. potatoes, rice, beans, corn, and grains) foodstuff that we use for energy, stored in liver and muscle as glycogen stores before an endurance event.

Carbohydrate loading - a process that elevates muscle glycogen stores before an endurance event.

Carcinogens - Substances that are capable of inducing cancerous changes in cells and/or tissue.

Cardiac - pertaining to the heart.

Cardiac Arrhythmia -an abnormal heart rate or rhythm.

Cardiovascular system - heart and blood vessels.

Carotene - a yellow to orange pigment that is converted into vitamin A in the body. There are several different forms, including alpha-, beta-, and gamma-carotene.

Carotenoids - a group of phytochemicals that act as antioxidants and includes the carotenes as well as some other substances.

CAT scan - computerized axial tomography scan. A computerized x-ray scanning procedure used to create a three dimensional picture of the body, or part of the body, for the purpose of detecting abnormalities.

Catatonia - a state in which an individual becomes unresponsive; a stupor.

Central nervous system(CNS) - the brain and spinal cord.

Cerebral - pertaining to the brain.

Chelation - a chemical process by which a larger molecule or group of molecules surrounds or encloses a mineral atom.

Chelation therapy - the introduction of certain substances into the body so that they will chelate, and then remove, foreign substances such as lead, cadmium, arsenic, and other heavy metals. Chelation therapy can also be used to reduce or remove calcium-based plaque from the linings of the blood vessels, easing the flow of blood to vital organs and tissues.

Chemotherapy - treatment of disease by the use of chemicals (such as drugs), especially the use of chemical treatments to combat cancer.

Chlorophyll - the pigment responsible for the green color of plant tissues. It can be taken in supplement form as a source of magnesium and trace elements.

Cholesterol - a crystalline substance found in soluble fat, which serves in the transporting and absorption of fatty acids. However, excess amounts can be a potential health threat.

Chromosome - any of the threadlike strands of DNA in the nuclei of all living cells that carry genetic information. There are normally forty-six chromosomes (twenty-three pairs) in all human cells, with the exception of egg and sperm cells.

Coenzyme - a molecule that works with an enzyme to enable the enzyme to perform its function in the body. Coenzymes are necessary in the utilization of vitamins and minerals.

Cold-pressed- a term used to describe food oils that are extracted without the use of heat in order to preserve nutrients and flavor.

Complete protein - a source of dietary protein that contains a full complement of the eight essential amino acids.

Complex carbohydrate - a type of carbohydrate that, owing to its chemical structure, releases its sugar into the body relatively slowly and also provides fiber. The carbohydrates in starches and fiber are complex carbohydrates. Also called polysaccharides.

C-reactive protein(CRP) - an indicator of inflammatory activity that is associated with increased risk of heart attack.

Coronary arteries - blood vessels that originate from the aorta and branch out to supply oxygen and fuel to the heart muscle.

Coronary prone - having several risk factors related to the development of heart disease.

Cortisol - stress hormone secreted by adrenal gland.

Creatine phosphate (CP) - energy rich compound that backs up ATP in providing energy for muscles.

Dementia - a permanent acquired impairment of intellectual function that results in a marked decline in memory, language ability, personality, spatial skills, and/or cognition (orientation, perception, reasoning, abstract thinking, and calculation). Dementia can be either static or permanent, and can result from many different causes.

Deoxyribonucleic Acid (DNA) - the source of the genetic code housed in the nucleus of the cell.

Diabetes Type II - a disease in which the ability of the body to use sugar is impaired and sugar appears abnormally in the urine. It is caused by a deficiency of insulin.

Diastolic pressure - lowest pressure exerted by blood in an artery; occurs during the resting phase (diastole) of the heart cycle.

Dieting - eating according to a prescribed plan.

Diuretic - tending to increase urine flow, or a substance that promotes the excretion of fluids.

DNA - see Deoxyribonucleic Acid.

Edema - retention of fluid in the tissues that results in swelling.

EEG - Electroencephalogram. A test used to measure brain wave activity.

Electrocardiogram (ECG) - A graphing recording of the electrical activity of the heart.

Electrolyte - solutions of ions (sodium, potassium) that conducts electric current.

Embolus - a loose particle of tissue, a blood clot, or a tiny air bubble that travels through the bloodstream and, if it lodges in a narrowed portion of a blood vessel, can block blood flow.

Endocrine system - the system of glands that secrete hormones into the bloodstream. Endocrine glands include the pituitary, thyroid, thymus, and adrenal glands, as well as the pancreas, ovaries, and testes.

Endorphin - one of a number of natural hormone-like substances found primarily in the brain. One function of endorphins is to suppress the sensation of pain, which they do by binding to opiate receptors in the brain.

Endurance - the ability to persist or to resist fatigue.

Enzyme - an organic catalyst that accelerates the rate of chemical reactions.

Epidemic - an extensive outbreak of a disease, or a disease occurring with an unusually high incidence at certain times and places.

Essential Fatty Acids - unsaturated fatty acids that are essential for health, but not produced by the body. EFA's are commonly found in cold-pressed oils, particularly oils extracted from cold-water fish and certain seeds.

Epinephrine (adrenaline) - hormone from the adrenal medulla and nerve endings of the sympathetic nervous system; secreted during times of stress and to help mobilize energy.

Exercise - means structured physical activity, but usually denotes any form of physical activity, exertion, effort, and so forth.

Fat-important energy source - stored for future use when excess calories are ingested.

Fat - soluble - capable of dissolving in the same organic solvents as fats and oils.

Fatigue - diminished work capacity, usually short of true physiological limits; real limits in short, intense exercise are factors within muscle pH and Calcium; in long-duration effort, limits are glycogen depletion or central nervous system fatigue caused, in part, by low blood sugar.

Fatty Acid - any one of many organic acids from which fats and oils are made.

FBS - fasting blood sugar. The level of glucose present in a blood sample drawn at least eight hours after the last meal.

Fiber - the indigestible portion of plant matter and an important component of a healthy diet. It is capable of binding to toxins and escorting them out of the body.

Fibrillation - rapid and uncoordinated contractions in the heart that can be life threatening.

Fitness - a combination of aerobic capacity and muscular strength and endurance that enhances health, performance, and the quality of health.

Flatulence - excessive amounts of gas in stomach or other parts of digestive tract.

Flavonoid - any of a large group of crystalline compounds found in plants. Also called bioflavonoid.

Flexibility - range of motion through which the limbs or body parts are able to move.

Free Radical - an atom or group of atoms with at least one unpaired electron. Because free radicals are highly reactive, they can alter the chemical structure of cells and may accelerate the progression of cancer and cardiovascular disease.

Functional Foods - foods that have been enriched or fortified with vitamins, herbs, or minerals to provide a health benefit beyond the product's traditional nutrients. For example- orange juice with calcium.

Gastritis - inflammation of the stomach lining.

Gastroenteritis - inflammation of the mucous lining of the stomach and the intestines.

Gastrointestinal - pertaining to the stomach, small and large intestines, colon, rectum, liver, pancreas, and gallbladder.

GERD - gastro esophageal reflux disease. Medical term for a syndrome characterized by frequent indigestion or heart burn.

Ghrelin - a hormone that helps regulate body weight and metabolism

Gland - an organ or tissue that secretes a substance for use elsewhere in the body rather than for its own functioning.

Globulin - a type of protein found in blood. Certain globulins contain disease-fighting antibiotics.

Glucose - basic carbohydrate energy source transported in blood; essential energy source for brain and nervous tissue.

Gluten - a protein found in many grains, including wheat, rye, barley, and oats.

Glycemic index - a measure of how rapidly a carbohydrate is digested and absorbed into the blood.

Glycogen - storage form of glucose; found in liver and muscles.

Heart Attack - death of heart muscle tissue that results when a therosclerosis blocks oxygen delivery to heart muscle; also called myocardial infarction.

Heart rate - Frequency of contraction, often inferred from pulse rate (expansion of artery resulting from beat of heart).

Heat stress - combination of temperature, humidity that leads to heat disorders such as heat cramps, heat exhaustion, or heatstroke.

Heavy Metal - a metallic element whose specific gravity (a measurement of mass as compared with the mass of water or hydrogen) is greater than 5.0. Some heavy metals, such as arsenic, cadmium, lead, and mercury, are extremely toxic.

Hemoglobin - the iron containing red pigment in the blood that is responsible for the transport of oxygen.

Hepatitis - a general term for inflammation of the liver. It can result from infection or exposure to toxins.

Herbal therapy - the use of herbal combinations for healing or cleansing purposes. Herbs can be used in tablet, capsule, tincture, or extract form, as well as in baths and poultices.

High-density lipoprotein (HDL) cholesterol - a carrier molecule that takes cholesterol from the tissue to the liver for removal; inversely related to heart disease.

Histamine - a chemical released by the immune system that acts on various body tissues. It has the effect of constricting the smooth bronchial tube muscles, dilating small blood vessels, allowing fluid to leak from various tissues, and increasing the secretion of stomach acids.

Homeopathy - a medical system based on the belief that "like cures like"—that is, the illness can be cured by taking a minute dose of a substance that, if taken by a healthy person, would produce symptoms like those being treated. Homeopathy employs a variety of plant, animal, and mineral substances in very small doses to stimulate the body's natural healing powers and to bring the body back into balance.

Hormone - one of numerous essential substances produced by the endocrine glands that regulate many bodily functions.

Hyperthermia - an alarming rise in body temperature that sets the stage for heat stress disorders.

Hyperglycemia - high blood sugar.

Hypertension - high blood pressure. Generally hypertension is defined as a regular resting pressure over 140/90.

Hypoglycemia - low blood sugar (glucose).

Hypotension - low blood pressure.

Hyponatremia - low sodium concentrations generally resulting from excess fluid intake or excess sweating without sodium replacement.

Hypothermia - life-threatening heat loss brought on by rapid cooling, energy depletion, and exhaustion.

Hypoxia - low oxygen

Idiopathic - term describing a disease of unknown cause.

Immune System - a complex system that depends on the interaction of many different organs, cells, and proteins. Its chief function is to identify and eliminate foreign substances such as harmful bacteria that have invaded the body. The liver, spleen, thymus, bone marrow, and lymphatic system all play vital roles in the proper functioning of the immune system.

Immunodeficiency - a defect in the functioning of the immune system. It can be inherited or acquired, reversible or permanent. Immunodeficiency renders the body more susceptible to illness of every type, especially infectious illnesses.

Infection - invasion of body tissues by disease-causing organisms such as viruses, protozoa, fungi, or bacteria.

Inflammation - a reaction to illness or injury characterized by swelling, warmth, and redness.

Insomnia - the inability to sleep.

Insulin - Pancreatic hormone responsible for getting blood sugar into cells.

Insulin resistance - a condition in which people produce adequate, or excess, insulin but have insulin receptors on muscle cells that have become insensitive to insulin and no longer stimulate muscle cells to take up glucose from the blood.

Interferon - a protein produced by the cells in response to viral infection that prevents viral reproduction and is capable of protecting uninfected cells from viral infection. There are different types of interferon, designated alpha, beta, and gamma.

Interleukin - any of a number of immune system chemicals manufactured by the body to aid in fighting infection.

Intravenous (IV) infusion - the use of a needle inserted in a vein to assist in fluid replacement or the giving of medication.

Ischemia - lack of blood to a specific area such as heart muscle.

Isoflavones - plant based compound with estrogen-like properties that are found primarily in soybeans. Isoflavones can act as a low-dose estrogens and can also lessen estrogen's effect on cells and skin layers, possibly reducing the risks of estrogen-related cancers.

IU - international unit. A measure of potency based on an accepted international standard. Dosages of vitamin A and E supplements, among others, are usually measuring international units. Because this is a measurement of potency, not weight or volume, the number of milligrams in an international unit varies, depending on the substance being measured.

Ketogenic diet - a diet that produces acetone or ketone bodies, or mild acidosis.

Lactase - an enzyme that converts lactose into glucose and galactose. It is necessary for the digestion of milk and milk products.

Lactic acid - a by-product of glycogen metabolism that also transports energy from muscle to muscle and from muscle to the liver; high levels in muscle poison the contractile apparatus and inhibit enzyme activity.

Lean body weight - body weight minus fat weight.

Lecithin - a mixture of phospholipids that is composed of fatty acids, glycerol, phosphorus, and choline or inositol. All living cell membranes are largely composed of lecithin.

Leptin - a hormone produced by fat cells that helps regulate body weight and metabolism.

Limbic system - a group of deep brain structures that, among other things, transmit the perception of pain to the brain and generate an emotional reaction to it.

Lipid - Fat

Lipoprotein - a fat-protein complex that serves as a carrier in the blood (e.g., high density lipoprotein cholesterol).

Lipoprotein lipase (LPL) - an enzyme in adipose tissue (also found in muscle). Its activity has been found to increase in the fat cells of obese people who lose weight.

Low density Lipoprotein (LDL) cholesterol - the cholesterol fraction that accumulates in the lining of the coronary arteries and causes atherosclerosis and ischemia.

Lutein - a phytochemical (one of carotenoids) found in kale, spinach, and other dark green leafy vegetables that is beneficial for the eyes. It may help protect against macular degeneration.

Lycopene - a phytochemical found in tomatoes that appears to afford protection against prostate cancer and to protect the skin against harm from ultraviolet rays.

Lymphadenopathy - enlargement of a lymph node or nodes as a result of the presence of a foreign substance or disease. This condition is often referred to as "swollen glands."

Metabolic rate - also called resting metabolic rate, this is the energy expenditure rate that occurs during quiet sitting and rest. It is estimated at 3.5 milliliters of oxygen per kilogram of body weight each minute (about 1.25 calories each minute for a 155 pound person) but varies slightly within and between individuals.

Metabolic syndrome - a clustering of metabolic abnormaliites including elevated blood pressure, triglycerides, and blood glucose, with central adiposity (waist circumference greater than 40 inches or 100 centimeters) and low HDL cholesterol.

Metabolism - energy production and utilization processes, mediated by enzymatic pathways.

Mineral - a micro-nutrient that is neither animal-nor plant based such as calcium, iron, potassium, sodium and zinc, which is essential to the nutrition of humans, animals, and plants.

Mitochondria - tiny organelles within cells; site of all oxidative energy production.

Motor neuron - nerve that transmits impulses to muscle fibers.

Motor unit - motor neuron and the muscle fibers that it innervates.

MRI - magnetic resonance image. A technique used in diagnosis that combines the use of radio waves and a strong magnetic field to produce detailed images of the internal structures of the body.

Muscle fiber types - fast twitch fibers are fast contracting but fast to fatigue; slow twitch fibers contract somewhat more slowly but are fatigue resistant.

Natural Foods - these foods are minimally processed and contain no artificial colors, flavorings, preservatives, or sweeteners.

Naturopathy - a form of healthcare that uses diet, herbs, and other natural methods and substances to cure illness. The goal is to produce a healthy body state without the use of drugs by stimulating innate defenses.

Neurogenic - training that influences the nervous system.

Neuron - nerve cell that conducts an impulse; basic unit of the nervous system.

Neurotransmitter - a chemical that transmits nerve impulses from one nerve cell to another. Major neurotransmitters include acetylcholine, dopamine, gamma-aminobutyric acid, norepinephrine, and serotonin.

Nucleic Acid - any of a class of chemical compounds found in all viruses and plant and animal cells. Ribonucleic acid(RNA) and deoxyribonucleic acid (DNA),which contain the genetic instructions for every living cell, are two principal types.

Nutraceutical - a food or nutrient based product or supplement designed and/or used for a specific clinical and/or therapeutic purpose.

Nutrition - provision of adequate energy (calories) as well as needed amounts of fat, carbohydrate, protein, vitamins, minerals, and water.

Obesity - excessive body fat (more than 20 percent of total body weight for men, more than 30 percent for women).

Organic Foods - the U.S. Department of Agriculture (USDA) strictly enforced proper production of these foods by using the following categories

- **"100 Percent organic"** - products included all organically produced(raw and processed) ingredients(excluding water and salt). The "100 percent organic" label may be used, as may the USDA organic seal. The organic certifying agent must be identified on the label, as must the seal.

- **"USDA Certified Organics"** - made with 95 percent or more organic ingredients. These foods may be labeled as "organic" and carry the USDA organic seal. The name of the certifying agent must appear on the label, although the seal is optional.

- **"Made with Organic Ingredients"** - foods may include 70 to 95 percent organic ingredients. Up to three of these organic ingredients may be listed on the primary display panel along with the "Made with Organic Ingredients" tag. The name of the certifying agent must be included; the USDA organic seal cannot be used.

-**Foods made with less than 70 percent organic content** can include the organic ingredients on the ingredient label. This term can be found in the informational panel on applicable products and identifying ingredients. It cannot be used on the primary display panel, however, and no seals can be used. Specific requirements to be certified organic vary slightly for different types of livestock, dairy and agricultural producers.

Osteoporosis - a disorder in which minerals leach out of the bones, rendering them progressively more porous and fragile.

Oxidation - the process of breaking down fuels (carbohydrate, fat, and protein) in the presence of oxygen to produce energy (ATP and heat) plus carbon dioxide (CO_2) and water (H_2O).

Peripheral nervous system - parts of the nervous system not including the brain and spinal cord.

Phenylketonuria (PKU) - an inherited disorder caused by a lack of enzyme necessary to convert the amino acid phenylalanine into another amino acid, tyrosine, so that excesses can be eliminated from the body. A buildup of excess phenylalanine in the blood can lead to neurological disturbances and mental retardation.

Phytochemical - any one of many substances present in fruits and vegetables. There are hundreds of phytochemicals, and more are being identified every day. Some appear to help protect the body against illness, including such serious diseases as cancer and heart disease.

Pituitary - a gland located at the base of the brain that secretes a number of different hormones. Pituitary hormones regulate growth and metabolism by coordinating the actions of other endocrine glands.

Physical fitness - the state of energy (aerobic) fitness or muscular (strength and power) fitness.

Placebo - a pharmacologically inactive substance, primarily used in experiments to provide a basis for comparison with pharmacologically active substances.

Plaque - a growth of cellular debris and low-density lipoprotein cholesterol that impedes blood flow in the arteries.

Progesterone - a hormone whose functions include preparing a woman's body for pregnancy in the second half of the menstrual cycle. Progesterone cream is used in hormone replacement therapy to prevent vaginal atrophy.

Prognosis - a forecast as to the likely course and/or outcome of a disorder or condition.

Protein - organic compound formed from amino acids; forms muscle tissue, hormones, and enzymes.

Pulse - the wave that travels down the artery after each contraction of the heart.

Radiation - energy that is emitted or transmitted in the form of waves. The term is often used as radioactivity; however, radioactivity is a specific type of radiation that comes from the decay of unstable atoms.

Rapid eye movement (REM) - a stage of sleep associated with dreams.

Relaxation response - proven method to achieve relaxation.

Ribonucleic acid (RNA) - a cellular compound that carries messages from the nucleus (DNA) to the rest of the cell (messenger RNA) or transfers amino acids to the ribosome for protein synthesis(transfer RNA).

Ribosome - a cellular organelle that synthesizes protein from amino acids.

RDA - an acronym for Recommended Daily Allowance or Recommended Dietary Allowance. The estimated amount of a nutrient, or calories, per day considered necessary for the maintenance of good health as determined by the U.S. food and Drug Administration.

Red Blood Cell - blood cell that contains the red pigment hemoglobin and transports oxygen and carbon dioxide in the bloodstream.

Saturated Fat - A fat that is solid at room temperature. Although most are of animal origin, some like coconut oil and palm oil come from plants. An excess of saturated fats in the diet may raise cholesterol levels in the bloodstream.

Seizure - a sudden, brief episode characterized by changes in consciousness, perception, muscular motion, and/or behavior. A convulsion is a type of seizure.

Serotonin - a neurotransmitter found principally in the brain that is considered essential for relaxation, sleep, and concentration.

Simple carbohydrate - a type of carbohydrate that, owing to its chemical structure, is rapidly digested and absorbed into the bloodstream. Glucose, lactose, and fructose are examples of simple carbohydrates.

Sorbic Acid - an organic acid used as a food preservative.

Steroid - one of a group of fat-soluble organic compounds with a characteristic chemical composition. A number of different hormones, drugs, and other substances, including cholesterol, are classified as steroids.

Stroke - an attack in which the brain is suddenly deprived of oxygen as a result of interrupted blood flow. If it continues for more than a few minutes, brain damage and even death may result.

Strength - ability of muscle to exert force.

Sublingual - literally, under the tongue, sublingual medications and supplements often look like tablets or liquids meant for swallowing, but they are designed to be held in the mouth while the active ingredient is absorbed into the bloodstream through the mucous membranes.

Syncope - temporary loss of consciousness; fainting.

Syndrome - a group of signs and symptoms that together are known or presumed to characterize a disorder.

Systemic - pertaining to the entire body.

Systolic pressure - highest pressure in arteries that results from contraction (systole) of the heart.

Tendon - tough connective tissue that connects muscle to bone.

Tension - the condition of being strained, stressed.

Testosterone - an anabolic (tissue building) hormone found in higher concentrations in males.

Thrombus - an obstruction in the blood vessel.

Topical - pertaining to the surface of the body.

Toxicity - the quality of being poisonous. Toxicity reactions in the body impair bodily functions and/or damage cells.

Toxin - a poison that impairs the health and functioning of the body.

Tremor - involuntary trembling.

Triglyceride - a fat consisting of three fatty acids and glycerol.

Type A Personality - A personality that tends to be impatient and aggressive. Persons with type A personalities tend to have stronger stress reactions and may be more susceptible to cardiovascular disease.

Type B Personality - A personality that tends to be relaxed and patient, and less reactive to stress. Those with type B personalities may be less prone to develop stress related illnesses such as high blood pressure and heart disease.

Unsaturated Fat - any of a number of dietary fats that are liquid at room temperature. Unsaturated fats come from vegetable sources and are good sources of essential fatty acids. Examples include flaxseed oil, sunflower oil, safflower oil, and primrose oil.

Urticaria - hives

Vaccines - a preparation administered to achieve immunity against a specific agent by inducing the body to make antibodies to that agent. A vaccine may be a suspension of living or dead microorganisms, or a solution of an allergen or viral or bacterial antigens.

Vegan - these products are derived solely from plant origin, excluding animal protein (such as meat, eggs, dairy products, or honey).

Vegetarian - foods derived from plant sources such as vegetables, fruits, grains, legumes, and nuts. May contain some animal protein, usually using egg or dairy products as ingredients.

Ventricle - chamber of the heart that pumps blood to the lungs (right ventricle) or to the rest of the body (left ventricle).

Vitamin - one of a group of organic substances essential in small quantities for life. For the most part, they must be supplied through the diet, since the body does not manufacture them.

Warm up - a pre-exercise activity used to increase muscle temperature and rehearse skills.

Water-soluble - capable of dissolving in water.

Weight training - progressive resistance exercise using weight for resistance.

Wellness - a conscious and deliberate approach to an advanced state of physical, physiological, and spiritual health.

White Blood Cell - a blood cell that functions in fighting infection and in wound repair.

Withdrawal - the process of adjustment that occurs when the use of a habit-forming substance to which the body has become accustomed is discontinued.

Work - product of force and distance

Work Capacity - the ability to achieve work goals without undue fatigue and without becoming a hazard to oneself or coworkers; also referred to as sustainable work capacity.

References and Recommended Readings

Balch PA. Prescription for Nutritional Healing. 4th ed. New York, NY: Avery Penguin Group; 2006. pp 3-807.

Going Green. Better Eating Starts With Knowledge, Food Glossary. The Palm Beach Post; 0930; 2007 pp.1.

Sharkey BJ, Gaskill SE. Fitness & Health. 6th ed. Champaign, IL: Human Kinetics; 2007.pp 1-400.

Index

high fructose corn syrup, 7, 10, 11, 28
hiking, 101
hormones, 7, 8, 83, 84, 142, 143, 145, 146, 149, 181, 187, 198, 200
Huperzine, 54, 88
hypertension, 20, 56, 78, 87, 96, 98, 124, 131, 167, 169, 183, 191

I

immune system, 68, 83, 97, 132, 190, 192
insomnia, 59, 60, 64, 67, 69, 77, 78, 91, 128, 141
insulin, 7, 116, 145, 186, 192
Interleukin-6, 21
intestinal disorders, 77

K

Kale, 25

L

LDL, 67, 75, 80, 175, 194
Leptin, 193
lipid, 66
lutein, 10
Lutein, 11, 194
lycopene, 11, 25

M

mackerel, 4, 61, 73
Magnesium, 13, 54, 60, 74
math games, 157

memory, 7, 5, 10, 11, 54, 62, 64, 67, 68, 72, 73, 75, 82, 83, 85, 86, 88, 89, 90, 91, 103, 110, 131, 132, 147, 155, 156, 159, 161, 165, 177, 186
mercury, 4, 5, 63, 190
metabolic rate, 137, 169, 194
metabolism, 14, 53, 56, 66, 72, 87, 97, 144, 145, 150, 183, 189, 193, 198
methylsulfonylmenthane, 85
minerals, 59, 185, 189, 196, 197
mitochondria, 15
Mixed Meal Day, 38, 39, 40
MRI, 153, 195
MSM, 55, 85, 86

N

naps, 142, 146, 147
Natural Foods, 17, 195
neuroendocrine system, 145
Neurotransmitter, 195
neurovascular, 7, 1, 2, 3, 7, 14, 21, 22, 24, 52, 57, 61, 66, 69, 71, 75, 78, 80, 82, 124, 147, 166, 167
Niacin, 66, 67, 68
Niacinamide, 66, 67
Nicotinamide, 66
Nicotinic Acid, 66
norepinephrine, 86, 97, 161, 196
nutrition, 1, 23, 35, 47, 115, 119, 146, 160, 168, 176, 178, 195
nuts, 2, 8, 11, 13, 30, 32, 33, 39, 40, 41, 50, 59, 67, 74, 81, 201

About the Author

Paul Winner, DO, FAAN, FAAP, FAHS is director of both the Premiere Research Institute and the Palm Beach Headache Center in West Palm Beach, FL., where he is also an attending neurologist at Palm Beach Neurology. In addition he is Clinical Professor of Neurology at Nova Southeastern University in Ft. Lauderdale, FL.

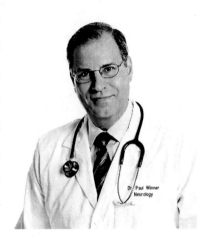

He earned his D.O. from the New York College of Osteopathic Medicine in Old Westbury in 1981, followed by a rotating internship in medicine at Suburban General Hospital in Norristown, PA. He completed residencies in Pediatrics and Neurology at the Albert Einstein College of Medicine in Bronx, NY. He then served as Neuromuscular Fellow in Neurology at Cornell University Hospital for Special Surgery in New York.

Dr. Winner is a member of several professional societies, including the American Medical Association and the American Osteopathic Association. He is Board Certified by the American Board of Psychiatry and Neurology with a special competence in Child Neurology. He is a Fellow of the American Academy of Neurology,

American Academy of Pediatrics, and the American Headache Society. He is Editor-in-Chief of Headache Update, Associate Editor of Headache, and a reviewer for several journals. He is also the President of the American Headache Society. He has been awarded Best Doctors in America in 2005-to present. He has also been awarded one of America's Top Physician.

Dr. Winner is an active presenter and author on the topics of Headache and Neurological Disorders. He has received major media attention and has participated as Investigator and Principal Investigator in numerous clinical studies.

Printed in the United States
115992LV00003B/14/P